A WEEK OF
BIG BREAKFASTS

THE DAILY FORMULA

7 parts protein

2 parts carbohydrate

2 parts fat

always eat your breakfast sweet!

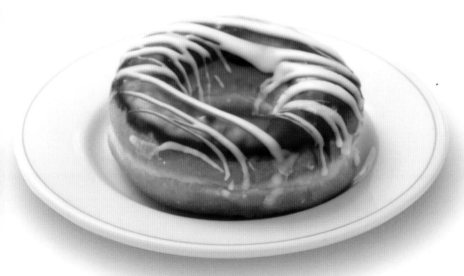

Here are 7 sample breakfasts to try.

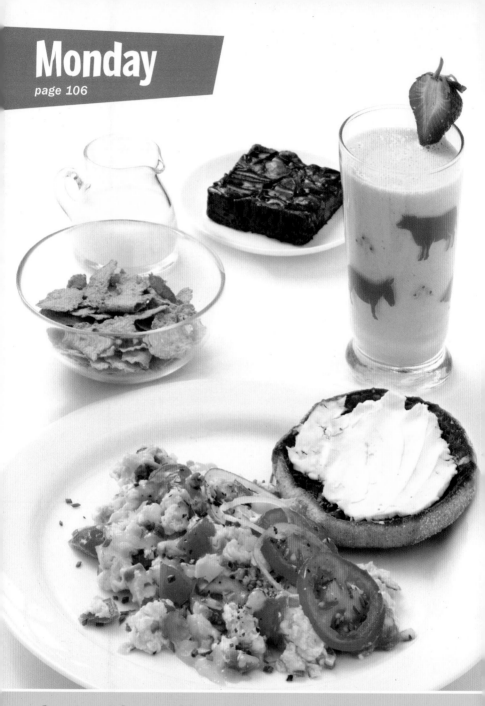

Country-style scramble, served with an English muffin and cream cheese, cereal with milk, a strawberry smoothie, and a gooey chocolate fudge brownie.

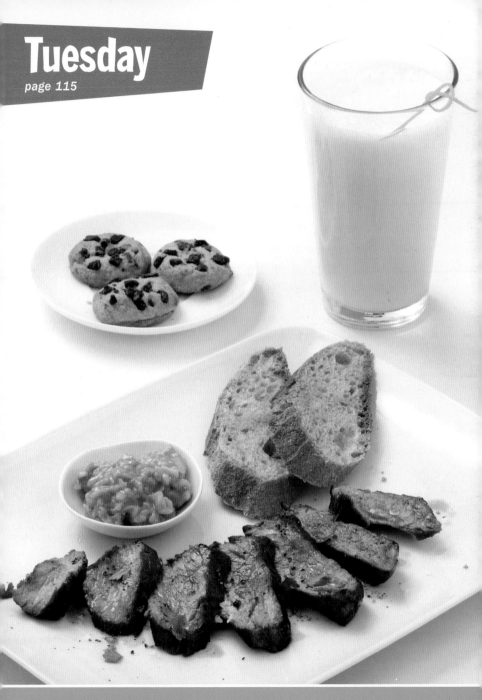

Broiled cowpoke steak with a piquant Parmesan spread, plus a hearty citrus shake, two slices of bread, and chocolate chip cookies.

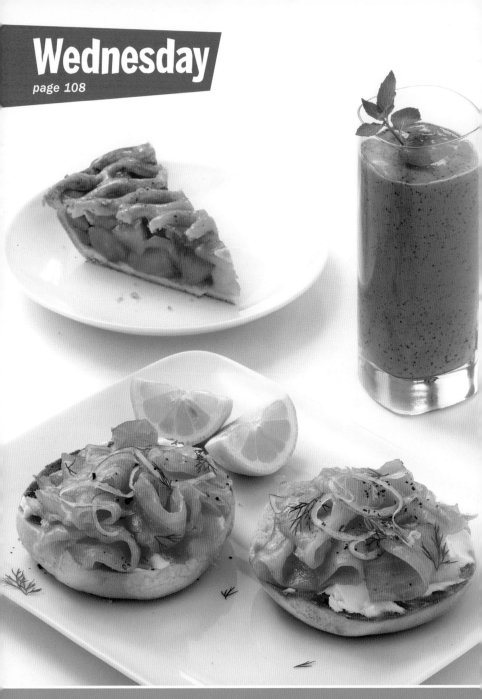

Smoked salmon on a cream cheese bagel, served with a blueberry smoothie and a warm slice of apple pie.

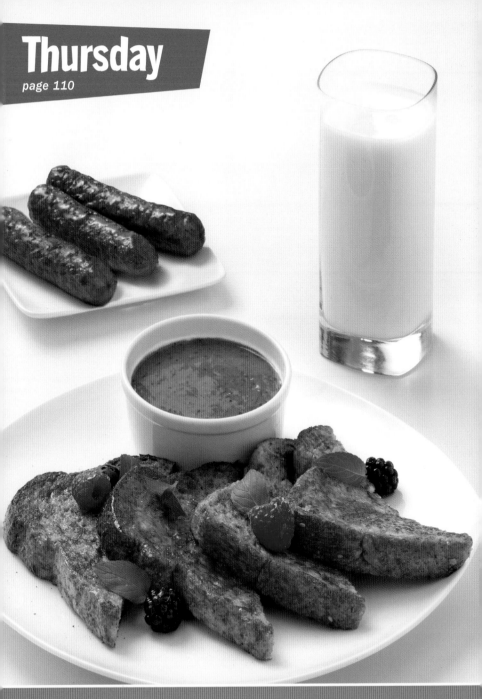

French toast topped with whipped yo-berry syrup and fresh berries, plus a side of turkey sausage, all washed down with a glass of low-fat milk.

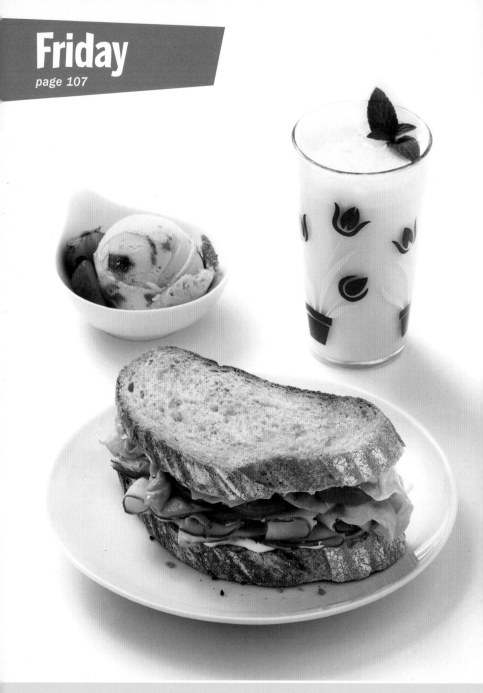

A toasted turkey and cheese sandwich, served with a rich banana shake and a dish of strawberry ice cream.

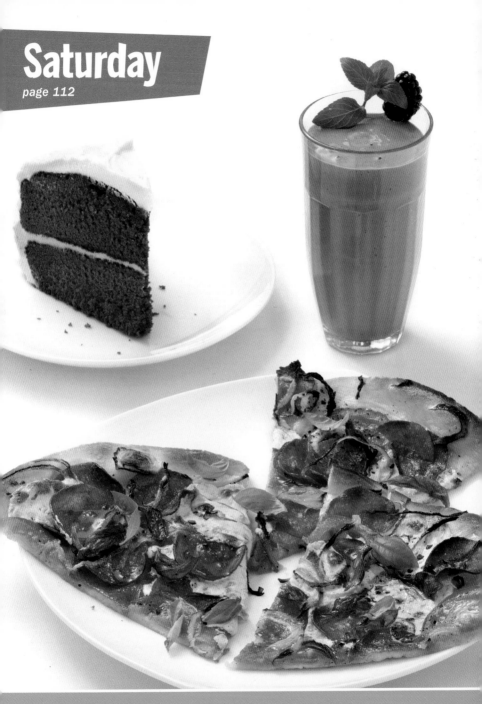

Pepperoni pizza topped with melted mozzarella, plus a blackberry smoothie and a sumptuous slice of red velvet cake.

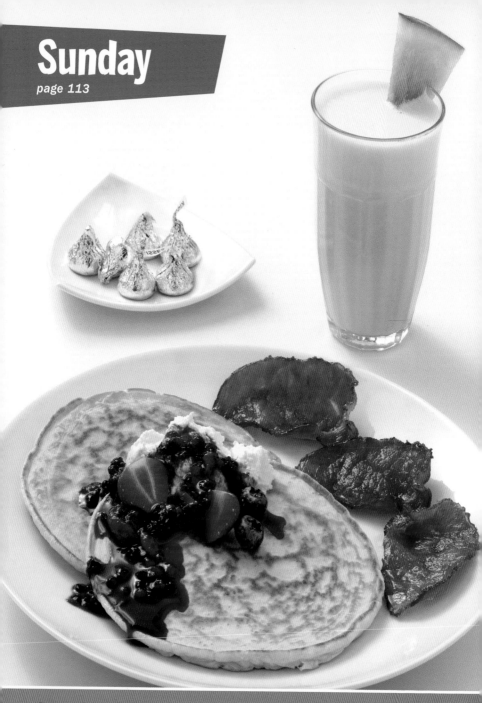

Pancakes and ricotta cheese drizzled with berry syrup, served with a side of crispy Canadian bacon, plus a watermelon smoothie and chocolate of your choice.

THE BIG BREAKFAST DIET

Eat Big Before 9AM, and Lose Big For Life

DANIELA JAKUBOWICZ, M.D.

WORKMAN PUBLISHING, NEW YORK

Library of Congress Cataloging-in-Publication Data is available.
ISBN 978-0-7611-5493-8

Book cover by Janet Vicario
Book interior by Sara Edward-Corbett
Cover illustration by Laurie Rosenwald

Workman books are available at special discounts when purchased in bulk for premiums and sales promotions as well as for fund-raising or educational use. Special editions or book excerpts can also be created to specification. For details, contact the Special Sales Director at the address below.

Workman Publishing Company, Inc.
225 Varick Street
New York, NY 10014-4381
www.workman.com

Printed in the United States of America
First printing December 2009
10 9 8 7 6 5 4 3 2 1

CONTENTS

RISE AND SHINE
TO LASTING
WEIGHT LOSS

Do you skip breakfast and eat almost nothing all day, only to go on an ice-cream bender at night? Do you eat constantly, unable to satisfy your hunger? Or maybe you try each new diet that comes along, do fine for a while, then get blindsided by cravings for sweets or starches.

If you're nodding in recognition, I know how you feel—I hear this over and over from the men and women who come to my office, desperate to lose weight. The hunger and cravings are common and frustrating scenarios—but they *can* be prevented. And I can help.

Fifteen years ago, while treating patients with metabolic conditions that often cause weight gain, including type 2 diabetes and polycystic ovary syndrome (PCOS, a common cause of female infertility), I made a discovery: When I tweaked their diets so that they ate certain types of foods at certain times—in effect, syncing food choices to the daily rhythm of specific hormones— they lost weight more quickly and easily.

Since then, I've successfully prescribed this program to many of my patients, as well as to new patients referred to me by their physicians—and I follow the program myself.

You're probably thinking, Come on. Losing weight is about eating less and moving more. Calories in and calories out.

But it isn't—and the science is there. In 2008, at the 90th annual meeting of the Endocrine Society, I stood in front of hundreds of my fellow endocrinologists and presented a clinical study of overweight women that demonstrated the effectiveness of my plan. Specifically, the study found that the women who followed it lost *almost five times as much weight* as women who followed a typical restrictive low-carbohydrate diet.

Yes, you read that right. This is a weight-loss plan that:

▶ revs up your metabolism,
▶ helps you burn more calories by day and more fat at night,
▶ allows you to enjoy your favorite foods—ice cream, cookies, pasta—and still lose weight,
▶ satisfies your hunger all day,
▶ crushes those diet-derailing cravings for sweets,
▶ gives you energy to burn,
▶ allows you to feel alert and refreshed, rather than sluggish and foggy, when you wake up,
▶ reduces your risk for serious health conditions such as type 2 diabetes and heart disease, and
▶ has reduced migraine occurrences among migraine sufferers.

The news gets better. You can have chocolate for breakfast. Or a dish of ice cream. Or a doughnut—plain, glazed, jelly, it doesn't matter, because you don't count calories on this plan.

But that's not all. You can *also* enjoy a cheese omelette with buttered toast and bacon, or a deli sandwich with mayo. On top of that, a fruit smoothie or a chocolate protein shake rounds out your meal.

On my plan, it's all about breakfast. A *big* breakfast. A breakfast similar to the one you might enjoy on a Sunday morning at your local diner. In fact, you can have a Sunday breakfast every day.

I know what you must be thinking. You don't have time to fix a huge meal before work. (I'll show you how.) You can't face food until lunchtime. (You'll soon get used to it.) There's no way you can lose weight on a 600-calorie breakfast that includes chocolate. (I promise, you can.)

In fact, many of my patients lose 25 pounds in 30 days on this plan, but better yet, they keep those pounds off. (If you have just 10 pounds to lose, you may reach your goal weight sooner; every body is different and loses weight at its own pace.) On my program, you don't get hungry. Best of all, you don't crave sweets and starches, because you're allowed—no, *required*—to eat them.

I know you're skeptical. Because you've probably starved and deprived yourself on countless diets with little to show for it. But stick with me here. As I said before, my plan is based on science, and I follow it myself. (Hey, I love chocolate, too!)

My program works because it accomplishes a feat that few other diets can: It allows you to control the addictive forces that compel you to binge on sweets and starches, simply by enjoying them early in the day. You can eat foods that are forbidden on other diets and still lose weight. You'll avoid the hunger that accompanies low-calorie diets, and you'll short-circuit carbohydrate attacks. Your energy will soar, your mood will brighten, and your skin will glow. Best of all, food will never rule your life again.

The science is basic. Its guiding principle is

Eat in sync with your body's natural rhythms.

BREAK THROUGH TO LASTING WEIGHT LOSS

The Big Breakfast Diet program works because it controls hunger and satisfies cravings for sweets and starches. It's also healthier than your typical low-carb diet because it allows you to eat more fiber- and vitamin-rich fruit. Ultimately, it works because rather than eating what you've been conditioned to expect to nosh on at certain times of the day (cereal for breakfast, a sandwich for lunch, lasagna for dinner, with snacks in between), you're giving your body what it needs when it needs it.

Natural rhythms, called circadian rhythms, influence your metabolism, body weight, hunger, and cravings. These rhythms dictate the body's hormonal "environment." Some hormones rule the body during the daylight hours, whereas others rule the night.

These hormones influence how the body uses carbohydrates and protein for fuel and how efficiently it burns body fat. It makes sense, then, that *eating the right foods at the right times* can diminish hunger and cravings for carbohydrates. No starving yourself, no cutting out certain foods. In fact, you'll eat quite well.

A hearty breakfast that includes plenty of protein speeds up your metabolism and controls your hunger for up to 14 hours. And its satisfying portion of carbohydrates, including sweets, boosts a hormone that regulates mood and cravings, addressing and controlling those afternoon and evening sugar and starch cravings *before* they kick in.

After this large, protein-packed breakfast, you probably won't be hungry for lunch, but please, eat anyway. This meal—a moderate amount of protein, fruit, and veggies—is tailored to your body's waning ability to use blood glucose for fuel as the day progresses, replacing high-sugar carbs with calorie-burning protein and fiber-packed, low-sugar vegetables and fruit.

If you follow the breakfast and lunch formulas to build your meals, you won't be hungry at the end of the day, because eating in sync throughout the day controls your hunger and cravings all night. However, a small dinner of low-sugar fruits and veggies and very little protein (if any) allows you to spend social time with your family and friends while maintaining the diet.

Adapt your sleep and exercise patterns to your body's natural rhythms and my eating plan becomes more powerful still. For example, exercise builds muscle; when you build muscle, you burn more calories and use more energy than you do storing body fat, even at rest and during sleep. However, exercising at the right time of day, when the body's hormonal landscape is primed for it, intensifies its benefits. In chapter 8, I'll give you the "prescription" for exercise that ends before the closing credits of your favorite TV show roll but gets your metabolism and weight loss moving.

So get ready to get healthy and have the body you want without giving up the foods you love. As the pounds melt away, you'll come to understand what my formerly overweight patients already know: The most important meal of the day can also be the sweetest.

THE
PROOF

MY BREAKFAST BREAKTHROUGH

I n my 2007 Big Breakfast study, women who began their day with a large, protein-packed breakfast that included a moderate amount of sweets and starches lost dramatically more weight than women who ate a very low carb breakfast. They continued to keep it off, too—without hunger or cravings.

BUT REALLY, WHAT KIND OF DOCTOR LETS YOU eat cookies at breakfast to lose weight?

One who's helped hundreds of overweight patients by prescribing this diet, that's who! And one who understands that permanent weight loss is less about *what* you eat than *when* you eat it. I know—a bite of chocolate at breakfast seems too good to be true—but the science of my plan is sound, solid, and very real.

When I graduated from medical school in 1973, the Atkins and Scarsdale diets were huge. Atkins was all about red meat, butter, and bacon—virtually no carbs and certainly no sweets. (It's since been updated, of course.) The Scarsdale Diet included some carbohydrates, but it allowed less than 1,000 calories a day.

THE SKINNY

Most calorie-controlled diets can lead to short-term weight loss, but they don't correct the underlying causes of gaining extra pounds: basic hunger and carbohydrate cravings. That's why most dieting frequently leads to more weight gain.

As an endocrinologist who treated many people with thyroid disorders and other health conditions that cause or contribute to weight gain, such as type 2 diabetes, I felt that neither diet approach was quite right. Why? Because I had read my endocrinology textbooks. Although I've simplified them here for easy digestion, these facts can be found in any of them:

▶ The human body's natural cycles, called circadian rhythms, regulate the hormones that control appetite, energy, mood, sleep, and metabolism.

▶ These hormone levels rise and fall depending on the time of day. One hormone, insulin, converts food to energy the body can use. This "fuel" is called blood glucose. (You'll learn more about insulin and other hormones in chapter 2.)

▶ Consuming a large amount of protein in the morning accelerates metabolism and controls hunger all day.

▶ Consuming a moderate amount of carbohydrates, including sweets, in the morning typically reduces urges for them later in the day.

I decided to see whether applying this textbook science could result in real-world weight loss. I began to counsel my overweight patients to eat a large, high-protein breakfast that included carbohydrates and sweets, followed by protein and low-sugar fruits and vegetables for lunch and dinner. It worked. My patients were elated and so was I. It felt good to be able to help people who, after many failures, were finally losing weight on a plan they could live with for life.

While treating patients, I also completed postgraduate work in neuroendocrinology (the study of communication between the brain and the endocrine system) and metabolic disease. Insulin's effects on type 2 diabetes and polycystic ovary syndrome (PCOS) particularly intrigued me. In collaboration with John Nestler, M.D., of Virginia Commonwealth University in Richmond, with whom I'd shared my early work, I began to test my plan in clinical studies on real people, particularly women with PCOS, which causes infertility, weight gain, and hair loss, among other symptoms.

In these studies, I learned more about how circadian rhythms affect appetite, hunger, and weight, and how the brain chemical serotonin acts as a natural tranquilizer and also regulates the craving for carbohydrates.

The 2008 Breakthrough

I began to present my research at endocrinology conferences around the world. In 2007, my team and I completed our most ambitious clinical study of my eating plan to date: an eight-month study of 94 overweight women with metabolic syndrome, a disorder involving the body's resistance to insulin. At the Endocrine Society's 2008 annual meeting, my team and I presented our study, in which we compared the effects of two food plans on weight loss, weight maintenance, hunger, and carb cravings.

The women who participated were divided into two groups. Both groups followed an overall very low carbohydrate (LCH) plan. But one group—let's call them the BB group, for Big

THE LCHs vs. THE BBs

Take a look at the diets of the 94 women in my study. The Big Breakfast Diet group consumed more calories each day than the Low Carb group, but their daily intake was front-loaded.

Group 1:
LOW CARBOHYDRATE DIET (LCH group)

▶ **BREAKFAST**
(250–350 CALORIES):
16 percent carbohydrates
28 percent protein
56 percent fat

▶ **LUNCH**
(450–550 CALORIES):
9 percent carbohydrates
39 percent protein
52 percent fat

▶ **DINNER**
(400–500 CALORIES):
12 percent carbohydrates
35 percent protein
53 percent fat

▶ **DAILY TOTAL**
(1,100–1,400 CALORIES):
12 percent carbohydrates
35 percent protein
53 percent fat

Group 2:
BIG BREAKFAST DIET (BB group)

▶ **BREAKFAST**
(610–850 CALORIES):
46 percent carbohydrates
37 percent protein
17 percent fat

▶ **LUNCH**
(350–400 CALORIES):
45 percent carbohydrates
38 percent protein
17 percent fat

▶ **DINNER**
(150–200 CALORIES):
15 percent carbohydrates
53 percent protein
32 percent fat

▶ **DAILY TOTAL**
(1,110–1,450 CALORIES):
41 percent carbohydrates
39 percent protein
20 percent fat

Adapted from the author's study "Effect of Diet with High Carbohydrate and Protein Breakfast on Weight Loss and Appetite in Obese Women with Metabolic Syndrome."

Breakfast group—ate a high-protein, high-calorie breakfast. Both groups stayed on the diet for four months to lose weight, and then shifted to weight maintenance for the next four months.

As I said, both groups consumed a very low amount of carbohydrates. The key difference: The BB group ate more carbohydrates, early in the day, and their typical breakfast contained roughly double the calories (for specific calorie and macronutrient breakdown for both plans, see page 5). A typical

----

DATA FROM MY
"BIG BREAKFAST" STUDY

Both groups lost weight . . . but only one group kept it off. During the first 16 weeks of the study, both groups lost a significant amount of weight. The LCH group lost 12.6 ± 2 kg (about 28 lb); the BB group, 10.6 ± 3 kg (about 23 lb). In the second 16 weeks, the BB group continued to lose weight, but the LCH group regained it. Look at the graph to see how they fared.

A high-carb, high-protein breakfast satisfies. We compared both groups' fullness, satiety, hunger, and prospective food consumption after their respective breakfasts. Compared to the LCH breakfast, the BB breakfast significantly diminished hunger and prospective food consumption, and enhanced fullness and satiety.

The BB group felt fuller all day. Compared to the LCH group, the BB group reported feeling significantly fuller after breakfast, after lunch, and for the rest of the day. The BB group reported that they felt more alert, too.

Carbohydrate cravings faded. Both groups completed a Food-Craving questionnaire. The results showed that overall craving for carbohydrates and starches had significantly decreased throughout the study for the BB group, but increased—and intensified—for the LCH group.

breakfast for them: a cup of milk, a turkey sandwich with cheese and mayo, an ounce of chocolate, and a protein shake.

The women on the traditional LCH plan, on the other hand, breakfasted on one egg, three slices of bacon, two teaspoons of butter on two slices of bread, and a cup of milk.

After four months, both groups had lost substantial weight. The LCH group lost an average of 28 pounds; the BB group, 23 pounds. We used a tool called the Food-Craving Inventory to

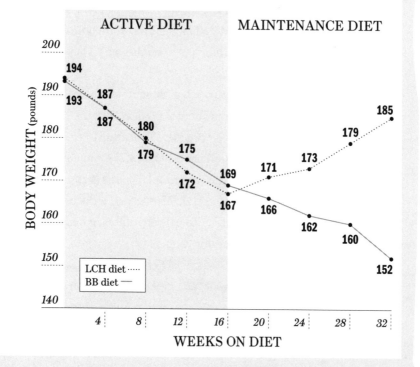

COMPARING THE TWO DIETS:
Weight Loss Outcomes in LCH Diet and BB Diet

ACTIVE DIET   MAINTENANCE DIET

BODY WEIGHT (pounds)

LCH diet ·····
BB diet —

WEEKS ON DIET

evaluate the frequency and intensity of both groups' cravings. The LCH group craved sweets and starches intensely, and often. The BB group barely experienced cravings at all.

Both groups then began the four-month weight-maintenance phase of the study. That's when things got interesting. The cravings for sweets and starches that had plagued the LCH group during the weight-loss phase rose even higher during the maintenance phase. Not surprisingly, 35 of the 46 women in the LCH group—76 percent—abandoned their plan, reporting that they simply could not resist their cravings for carbohydrates. When they returned to their old eating habits, they regained, on average, 18 pounds.

How did the BB group fare? Well, they continued to lose weight, shedding an additional 17 pounds. Better yet, only 4 of the 48 of the BB group—8 percent—abandoned the plan. The remaining 44 women continued it. They felt too good not to! Best of all, their craving for carbs was "in remission." They felt in control.

At the end of the eight months, after the maintenance period, the LCH group lost an average of about 9 pounds. But the BB group lost an average of nearly 40 pounds. That translated to an average body mass loss of 4.5 percent for the LCH group, and a 21.3 percent average loss for the BB group! The BB group was ecstatic about their weight loss, and thrilled to find a doctor who believed that they were "addicted" to carbohydrates, a belief that many of them had harbored for years.

You may wonder if the Big Breakfast Diet is as simple and satisfying as it sounds. My answer: an emphatic *yes*. If you keep losing and regaining the same 15, 20, or more pounds, there are probably a couple of things going on. First, overweight people frequently eat "out of sync," or against the body's natural rhythms. Second, they are frequently caught in a cycle of hunger and addiction, a phenomenon I call "Fat Brain." These two intertwine—one reinforces the other.

PROBLEM #1
Eating Out of Sync

If you've struggled with your weight for a long time, you probably blame your diet failures on a lack of willpower. Let me tell you, willpower has nothing to do with it. I'd wager that the problem isn't what you eat, it's when you eat it. Our circadian rhythms regulate our eating patterns. In simple terms, our eating patterns are screwed up. Think of jet lag, only with food.

Most overweight people become out of sync because they either skip breakfast or they eat too little in the morning. They go against their body's actual needs (fuel in the morning) and make up for it by over-fueling later.

When your body awakens from its eight-hour slumber, it is primed to seek food. Your metabolism is revved up, and levels of certain hormones (cortisol and adrenaline) are at their highest. Your brain needs energy (glucose) immediately.

If you don't break your eight-hour fast or you eat too little, your brain needs to find another source of fuel. So it activates an emergency system that pulls energy from muscle and destroys muscle tissue in the process. Then when you eat later, the body and brain are still in high-alert mode, so the body saves energy from the food as fat.

Compounding the problem, serotonin levels are highest in the morning. This means that you're least likely to crave sweets and starches when you first wake up, and you may not feel much like eating. But as the day wears on, serotonin levels dip and the

DO YOU EAT
OUT OF SYNC?

You already know that skipping breakfast can actually make you gain weight. But if you're overweight, you likely exhibit one or more of these *other* self-defeating eating behaviors. Check off those that describe the way you typically eat.

☐ **YOU EAT BREAKFAST BUT SKIMP ON PROTEIN.** If you're like most overweight people, breakfast—if you eat it—consists of carbohydrates such as bagels and muffins. When you eat a breakfast of almost pure carbs, your blood sugar and insulin levels spike. Once that blood sugar is used up, the excess insulin in your blood makes you hungry—typically for chocolate and other sugary carbohydrates.

What your body's morning hormonal landscape favors is protein. Eggs, low-fat dairy products, and other protein-rich foods satisfy hunger in the morning and last longer than carbohydrates do. Also, your body must work harder to convert proteins to blood glucose. This extra effort raises metabolism. In fact, eaten in the morning, proteins can increase metabolism (fat burning) from 20 to 30 percent. By contrast, carbs raise metabolism by only 5 to 10 percent.

cravings kick in. If you eat these foods, brain serotonin rises, and you begin to associate good feelings with them. This connection between carbs and calm creates an addictive cycle.

People who skip breakfast or engage in other out-of-sync eating behaviors (see box above) set themselves up for metabolic disaster. Their metabolism sputters. They're plagued by midafternoon fatigue and/or moodiness, so they rev up or unwind with candy bars and sugary coffee drinks. Their bodies burn less of what they eat as fuel and store more of it as body fat. Their bodies lose muscle and gain fat—lots of it.

☐ **YOU FOLLOW CRASH DIETS.** Yes, starvation diets cause rapid weight loss. But most of this lost "weight" is muscle, not fat.

Muscle burns more calories than fat. That means, when you lose muscle, your body needs fewer calories to maintain its current weight. In short, the more muscle you lose, the fewer calories you burn. That's how many overweight people gain weight on as little as 900 calories a day.

Besides, it's impossible to follow crash diets forever. Before long, your hunger and cravings return full force. You give in to "forbidden" foods, return to your poor eating habits, and regain the weight you lost—and more.

☐ **YOU EXPERIENCE "SUNSET DEPRESSION."** As the day wanes, serotonin levels fall and trigger low mood and an irresistible urge for carbs, especially if you're on a low-calorie or low-carbohydrate diet. That pastry or candy bar will ease your sunset depression, but since insulin's efficiency is on the wane, that energy will never reach your muscle cells. As a result, you'll "wear" it as fat.

☐ **YOU OVEREAT AT NIGHT.** If you're a night eater, like many of my patients, you likely consume too few calories and/or carbohydrates during the day. Overeating at night, especially carbohydrates, undermines the body's fat-burning mode.

INSULIN RESISTANCE
When the "Hunger Hormone" Runs Amok

Most overweight people are *insulin resistant*. With insulin resistance, the number of cell wall receptor sites (which allow glucose to pass through the wall to be converted to energy) is significantly reduced, therefore, the normal amount of insulin secreted by the pancreas can't get glucose into muscle cells. Because of the reduced number of receptor sites, glucose is

WHAT IS
INSULIN RESISTANCE?

When you have this metabolic disorder, your muscle, fat, and liver cells have trouble using the insulin made by your pancreas.

Imagine insulin as a key that opens tiny "doors" on the outside of cells. These doors are called receptors. Insulin "unlocks" these receptors (actually attaches to the cells). With the doors unlocked by insulin, glucose (blood sugar) can enter the cells and be converted to energy.

With insulin resistance, the cells may not have enough doors, or there may be something wrong with the doors themselves. Also, there might be a defect in how insulin attaches to the receptors.

The pancreas tries to keep up with the body's demand for insulin by producing more. In time, however, the pancreas cannot keep up, and excess glucose builds up in the bloodstream. Many people with insulin resistance have high blood levels of glucose *and* high blood levels of insulin.

While insulin resistance tends to run in families, excess weight also contributes to this condition because excess body fat interferes with muscles' ability to use insulin. A sedentary lifestyle interferes further.

Insulin resistance promotes:
► Easier weight gain,
► More hunger in people who are overweight or obese, compared to those of normal weight,
► Greater carbohydrate craving,
► Reduced feeling of satiety,
► Blunted postprandial (after-meal) increase of brain serotonin, correlated with increased carbohydrate craving,
► Poor adherence to diets, and
► Rapid regain of lost weight.

denied entry to the cells, so it is carried to the liver via the bloodstream. Once it is in the liver, this excess glucose is converted to fat and stored throughout the body.

A nasty consequence of insulin resistance is that it causes constant hunger, particularly for carbohydrates. Since your body can't properly convert food to energy, it thinks it's starving and demands more food, which leads to weight gain. As your body's ability to use insulin wanes and your weight goes up, your body further loses its ability to process food correctly, which leads to putting on even more extra pounds.

In fact, insulin resistance is at the root of carbohydrate addiction, which develops if your pancreas releases too much insulin after you eat sweets and starches. (Researchers call this condition postprandial reactive hyperinsulinemia.) Having too much insulin results in too strong an impulse to eat, too often, and a body that too readily stores food energy as fat.

All too often as well, overweight people with undiagnosed insulin resistance go on low-calorie diets that treat the symptom of their disorder—extra pounds—but not the insulin resistance itself. Even if they lose weight, carbohydrate "withdrawal" kicks in, and they regain the lost weight and often more.

Insulin resistance also threatens your health. When you're insulin resistant, the cells in your muscles, nervous system, and organs start to reject the high levels of insulin in your blood. Since the blood sugar cannot easily enter the cells where it's needed, much of the food energy is shuttled into the fat cells and you gain weight. Over time, as high insulin levels continue, even your fat cells can shut down and the glucose becomes trapped in the bloodstream, which can lead to type 2 diabetes.

Insulin resistance is also a hallmark of the metabolic syndrome, which is characterized by excess belly fat, elevated blood pressure, and an unhealthy imbalance in blood fats (high triglycerides, low levels of "good" HDL cholesterol, and high levels of "bad" LDL cholesterol). This cluster of symptoms raises the risk of developing atherosclerosis (hardening and narrowing of the arteries), heart attack, stroke, type 2 diabetes, and other diseases.

PROBLEM #2
"Fat Brain"

Can't stomach the thought of food in the morning? Ever experienced an irresistible urge for chocolate, sweets, or other carbs in the midafternoon or at night?

You're likely to have what I call "Fat Brain." The defining characteristics of this condition are:

▶ an aversion to breakfast, the result of eating out of sync, and
▶ a lust for sweets and starches that typically begins at around 3 P.M. and continues into the evening.

Here's the reason: Beginning in midafternoon, when the sunlight starts to fade and serotonin levels fall, your body craves certain foods in order to make up for the drop in serotonin. Foods such as chocolate, cake, ice cream, and sugary cereal imitate the "feel-good" power of this brain chemical.

Scientists have long debated whether humans can be addicted to carbohydrates, as they can to alcohol or drugs. Although the jury's still out, preliminary research suggests that it's possible. What many researchers do agree on is that carbohydrates, if not truly addictive, have addictive characteristics.

Sweets and starches raise the level of insulin in your blood. These elevated insulin levels facilitate the entry of the amino acid tryptophan to the brain. Once in the brain, tryptophan is converted to . . . serotonin. Are you beginning to see the connection?

Serotonin also modulates addictive impulses toward food, especially carbohydrates. Restricting carbs lowers serotonin, making the brain cry out for sweets.

Compared to people of a normal weight, overweight people tend to experience more dramatic daily oscillations of serotonin. At daybreak their levels of serotonin tend to be abnormally

THE FAT BRAIN CYCLE

7:00 A.M.: "BREAKFAST—YUCK!" When you wake up in the morning, you're not hungry. In fact, the thought of food makes you a little sick.

3:30 P.M.: "MUST . . . HAVE . . . CHOCOLATE." You obsess about the jar of chocolate kisses on your coworker's desk, or the honey bun in the office vending machine. You try to fight the craving, in the face of your afternoon "crash," caused by your brain's falling serotonin levels. Your good intentions crumble like a cookie.

3:31 P.M.: "AHH." Once you eat those kisses, or the honey bun, your brain is flooded with serotonin. Your sadness, moodiness, or anxiety disappears, and is replaced by calm and tranquility.

10:33 P.M., BEDTIME: "WHY DID I EAT THAT?!" Once serotonin reaches high levels in the brain, the cravings vanish, but the guilt kicks in. All too often, the cravings resurface later in the evening. (If only you'd eaten a large, protein-packed breakfast!)

7:00 A.M.: "I WILL NOT EAT BAD FOODS TODAY, NO MATTER WHAT." You awaken, and with your brain bathed in serotonin, you vow to withstand temptation today. (And what do you mean, "bad foods"?) But you're still not hungry, so you skip breakfast, and the cycle begins anew.

elevated—that's the reason they're not hungry for breakfast. At sunset their serotonin falls and the carb cravings kick in. That, in a nutshell, is Fat Brain.

Over time, you get into a rhythm: You skip breakfast, your serotonin plummets, you feel lousy, you eat sweets and starches to feel better, your insulin levels rise, your brain serotonin rises, and your mood brightens. The problem: You're perpetuating a vicious circle. The more you turn to sweets and starches to feel better, the more you associate these foods with positive feelings.

This is the essence of addiction. In fact, some research suggests that just as alcoholics turn to liquor to feel better, overweight people self-medicate with sweets and starches. Of course, the "medicine" hurts more than it helps. Fat Brain inevitably leads to more and more weight gain. What's next? A diet, of course. And when you have Fat Brain, restricting calories and carbohydrates is the worst thing you could possibly do.

DIET AND EXERCISE DON'T TREAT
FAT BRAIN

Most weight-loss experts tell overweight people that all it takes to lose weight is to eat less and exercise more. True—but such a simple solution does not factor Fat Brain into the equation.

Rosa, one of my patients, is a clear example of Fat Brain. Overweight even as a child, she rarely ate breakfast. Not only did she not want to eat in the morning, she actually got nauseated at the thought. So she skipped it. And lunch. But by 4 P.M. Rosa underwent a transformation: She was restless and felt a mixture of sadness and anxiety and an enormous desire for sweets.

DIETING
The Fast Track to Fat Brain

Some experts, me included, suspect that these abnormal oscillations of serotonin in the brain are the root of carb addiction. It would follow, then, that a weight-loss plan designed to manage serotonin surges and dips will help control the constant craving for sweets and starches.

Once you understand this, it's easy to see that the standard advice of most weight-loss experts—"eat less"—is useless. It's useless because it does nothing to treat the irresistible cravings for sweets and starches that plague most people with weight problems. In the face of this addiction, "dieting" isn't the answer. Unless you take steps to control it, you will always be held hostage by it.

The good news: You can control Fat Brain.

This craving, which she experienced like clockwork every afternoon, was stronger than her sincere desire to eat well and lose weight. Every afternoon, she gave in to her craving for sweets, and felt peaceful—for a moment. Then, those feelings of calm and well-being were washed away by a tidal wave of guilt: She'd broken her diet *again*.

Rosa was beyond frustrated. Every morning, after a night of bingeing on sweets and starches, she vowed to do better—and skipped breakfast. Every afternoon, the cravings tormented her, she gave in, and the guilt and self-loathing returned. The worst part was, although she was always on a diet, she was getting heavier by the day.

The "cure" for Fat Brain isn't counting calories and cutting out food groups. It's a way of eating that controls the twin causes of obesity: hunger and addiction. The Big Breakfast Diet does that.

The Big Breakfast Diet is more than a diet. It's a *strategy*. And that strategy is to control the forces that push you toward cookies, ice cream, chips, and other high-carbohydrate foods. On this plan, you enjoy carbs when your body is best able to use them as fuel. Few diets allow you to eat the high-calorie, high-carbohydrate foods that contributed to your weight problems to begin with. That's because they overlook a simple fact: Sweets and starches are needed to maintain the brain's serotonin levels, and, if they're eaten *at the right time of day,* when the body's hormonal environment can make the best use of them, the addiction can be controlled.

Research, including my own, has shown that eating carbohydrates or sweets in the morning prevents the moodiness and carb cravings of the afternoon by maintaining the brain's serotonin levels all day long. (See page 35 for more.) The calm and well-being that occur when we eat sweets and starches in the afternoon does not occur in the morning. You'll simply feel that you've eaten a starch or a sweet. But you'll be breaking the connection between eating carbs and good feelings. Eat this way for a while, and you'll suspect that someone pulled out your sweet tooth while you slept!

You'll also learn to eat those foods that promote *satiety,* the technical term for "feeling full" after you eat. This full, satisfied feeling plays a critical role in losing weight or maintaining weight loss. You'll learn more about satiety, and which foods most satisfy, in chapter 4.

Imagine seeing a food that routinely derails your diet— fresh-baked bread, pizza, a plate of brownies—and not feeling the urge to inhale it. On my plan, this is what you can expect. You'll be able to see it, note it, and pass it by (or, okay, you can grab it for tomorrow's breakfast). Your cravings will simply fade away. Control the addiction and you will be able to control your weight for life.

But you don't have to take my word for it. Listen to a few of my patients.

THE BIG BREAKFAST DIET SUCCESS STORIES
I'm FINALLY Losing Weight!

ROSA, 28:

"I'm finally in control of my eating. My eating doesn't control me."

I'd been overweight all my life, always the heaviest girl in my class. My worried mother took me to doctors and nutritionists, who put me on diets. They never worked. By the age of 17, I was 5'3" and 165 pounds. I'd lose weight, but before long, I'd give in to my favorite foods—chocolate, waffles, ice cream, and chips— and gain it all back.

Diet and binge, lose and gain. That was my pattern, and there seemed no way out. At 22, I dieted down to 170 pounds, and lost 15 more before I married at 24. I didn't consume more than 800 calories a day. A few months after my wedding, still on my restrictive diet, I got pregnant.

My OB/GYN told me to start eating, and I took his advice to the extreme. By my eighth month of pregnancy, I'd gained 55 pounds (the average gain during pregnancy is 25 to 35 pounds) and my blood pressure rose to dangerous levels. Three weeks before my due date, even medication couldn't lower my blood pressure; my life was in danger, and so was my baby's. My daughter was delivered by emergency C-section. Luckily, both of us were fine, but soon after delivery, I was 210 pounds.

Back to dieting. I tried every plan out there. When they failed, I returned to my starvation diet. Sure, I lost weight—three months after delivery, I weighed 180 pounds. But inevitably, I'd binge on sweets and starches, and the pounds piled back on.

At 27, I weighed 195 pounds. I cried to my cousin Isabel, who was in great shape. She told me about Dr. Jakubowicz and the Big Breakfast Diet. She'd been following the diet since the birth of her child six years ago and had lost 25 pounds. I took another look at Isabel's fit body and made an appointment.

After my evaluation, Dr. Jakubowicz told me I was overweight for one reason: I was addicted to carbohydrates. Break the addiction, she said, and I'd lose the weight. Then she put me on her eating plan.

It was tough to get used to eating in the morning—I'd never been a breakfast eater. But on the program, I ate a sandwich (I like ham and cheese on a roll), a cup of yogurt, a glass of lactose-free milk (I'm lactose intolerant), and a piece of cake. I thought, "There's no way I can lose weight eating all this." After that huge breakfast, I wasn't hungry for the rest of the day. But I always ate my grilled chicken or steamed fish, veggies, and fruit for lunch, and my stew for dinner.

I lost weight slowly—years of yo-yo dieting had damaged my metabolism—but I did lose. In two months I'd lost 12 pounds. My energy was high, my mood bright, and the terrible cravings that used to compel me to eat throughout the night were simply gone.

In another 18 months I lost 30 more pounds. I now weigh 153 pounds and look like a different woman. I feel different, too. My weight had always affected my self-esteem. I'd been willing to starve and take weight-loss drugs to be thin. My husband told me later that I looked sick—my face was so drawn and thin, he said, he was terrified I might die. Now I'm healthy and happy. My face isn't pinched with hunger anymore. I eat well, and I lose weight. My goal weight is 145 pounds, and when I get there, I will eat this way for life. No more yo-yo dieting for me. After being heavy and hungry my entire life, I'm finally in control—my eating doesn't control me.

JANET, 30:

"There's simply no better way to eat."

I started to gain weight at age 8, when my grandmother, who equated eating with love, began to take me to a local fast-food restaurant every afternoon. My "snack"—a large burger, large fries, and milkshake—was more than a meal for a hungry man. Yet I'd eaten lunch at school, and ate a hearty dinner later.

After a few months, hooked on greasy fast food and sugary soda, I gained weight and kept gaining. At age 16, I stood 5'3" and weighed 170 pounds, and I packed on 20 more pounds by the end of my freshman year in college.

At 21, taking a now banned weight-loss medication, I lost 35 pounds in a year. The drug made me edgy, so I stopped taking it—and ballooned to 215 pounds over the next three years.

On a popular low-carbohydrate diet, I dropped 63 pounds in 18 months—I weighed less than I did at 16. But my eating took a dark turn. Thrilled with my weight loss, I was determined to lose more. In the late afternoon, overwhelmed with sadness and anxiety, I'd polish off huge quantities of pizza, cheeseburgers, and ice cream.

While I ate, I felt exquisite calm. Afterward, overwhelmed by shame, I'd vomit up what I'd eaten or take laxatives and diuretics. The constant vomiting made my throat sore. I had developed bulimia.

Terrified, I forced myself to eat "normally" to restore my health and get to a healthy weight. "Normal," for me, meant no breakfast, a tiny portion of grilled chicken with salad and fruit for lunch, and a sandwich for dinner—less than 1,200 calories a day. Bulimia, however, destroys the metabolism: In less than a year I gained 70 pounds, tipping the scales at 225.

Desperate, I sought help from Dr. Jakubowicz, who placed me on the Big Breakfast Diet plan. In the morning I ate a huge deli-style roast beef or turkey sandwich with cheese and mayo, a chocolate protein shake, and a doughnut. I could have skipped lunch, but I ate my protein, veggies, and fruit. By midafternoon I still wasn't hungry, not even for frozen yogurt, which I typically craved around that time of day. Best of all, my urge to binge and purge faded. I haven't done either in four years now.

In my first year on the Big Breakfast Diet plan, I lost 56 pounds, and 20 more over the next three years. Now at 154 pounds, I'm not model thin, but I'm healthy and happy. I eat more than I ever have—including all the foods I love—and the pounds continue to slip off. Even when I reach my goal weight, I'll continue on the Big Breakfast Diet. For me, there's simply no better way to eat.

STEPHEN, 32:
"I'm sticking with this for life."

A heavy kid, I grew into a heavy adult. At 29 I weighed 260 pounds—way too much, even at 6'1". I'd tried every diet out there, but my pattern never changed: I'd lose the weight, then put it all (and more) back on in a matter of months.

In hindsight, I can see why. First, I didn't eat breakfast—I just wasn't hungry in the morning. (I've since learned that skipping breakfast slowed my metabolism.) Right before noon, tired and dizzy from lack of food, I'd scarf down a doughnut and a cup of sugary coffee to help me focus on my work. Lunch was a large burger and fries, a sugary soda, and a small ice cream. By 5 P.M., famished, I'd wolf down a couple of jelly doughnuts and more soda to hold me until dinner.

I'd get home from work at 6 P.M., starving—those doughnuts and soda didn't even put a dent in my hunger. I'd pick up the phone and order a pizza and a two-liter bottle of soda. While I waited for "dinner" to arrive, I scarfed chips or cookies. After all this heavy, sugary, carbohydrate-packed junk, I snacked all night long: more cookies, ice-cream sandwiches, whatever.

By my 31st birthday I weighed 290 pounds. Discouraged and frustrated, I confided in my mother. She did some research and found Dr. Jakubowicz. I made an appointment the same day. I was sick of being fat and ready to get healthy.

Dr. Jakubowicz gave me a battery of tests and a full evaluation, then put me on the Big Breakfast Diet. It felt strange to eat breakfast at first, but I got used to it. I started the day with a thick roast-beef-and-cheese sandwich on a roll, a fruit smoothie, and a chocolate bar. My before-lunch dizziness vanished—and so did my appetite. I could have skipped lunch, but dutifully ate my lean protein, garden salad, and fruit. I didn't miss my midafternoon doughnuts or ice cream—my hunger had simply evaporated. Dinner might be a salad or vegetable stew. Although that's a pretty small meal for a guy like me, I just wasn't hungry. Immediately, the weight poured off, and my energy levels went through the roof, especially in the morning.

I've followed this plan for nearly a year, and have lost 70 pounds. I now walk after work, and I'm lifting weights to gain strength and lose body fat. I feel better—and look better—than I ever have in my life. I still get to eat pizza, hamburgers and French fries, ice cream, and cookies. I just eat them in the morning. The Big Breakfast plan works. I'm sticking with this for life.

ARLENE, 31:
"Even with PCOS, I lost weight—and gained a baby."

From my first period, at age 11, my cycles were irregular. By 16 I hadn't menstruated in a year, and carried 25 extra pounds on my 5'3" frame. A doctor prescribed birth control pills to regulate my cycle and advised me to eat less and exercise more.

The pills did regulate my cycle, but they added 10 more pounds to my 185-pound body. But I can't blame the pills. My diet was atrocious. I didn't eat breakfast but made up for it later in the day: a drive-through lunch, sweets in the midafternoon, more fast food for dinner, peanuts in front of the TV, and ice cream before bed.

Several years later I stepped on the scale and gasped: I weighed 245 pounds. Worse, my wedding was just months away. Determined, I began yet another diet. Four months later I reached 200 pounds, and I got down to 190 before the wedding.

After five years of marriage, however, I'd reexpanded to 220. My husband loved me heavy or thin, though, and we decided to start a family. I stopped the pills before Christmas. By Valentine's Day, I hadn't gotten my period. I rushed to the store for a home-pregnancy test. Negative. I got my period a week later, but the next didn't arrive for two more months. How would I get pregnant when my periods were so messed up? My doctor said he couldn't help: We hadn't yet been trying for a year.

Fast-forward a year. No pregnancy. I switched doctors. The new one found cysts in my ovaries, diagnosed me with polycystic ovarian syndrome (PCOS), and prescribed a fertility drug. After a year, still no pregnancy. We tried fertility shots and artificial insemination three times. My last option: in vitro fertilization.

Depressed by our six-year quest to start a family, I'd ballooned to 230 pounds. That's when a friend gently suggested that perhaps my weight was affecting my fertility. I read up on the link between fertility and obesity. That's when I made an appointment with Dr. Jakubowicz.

After confirming my PCOS diagnosis, Dr. Jakubowicz put me on the Big Breakfast Diet to enhance my body's sensitivity to insulin and improve my odds of ovulation and conception. She also prescribed diabetes medicine for my condition.

I started the day with a huge breakfast: two chocolate protein shakes, a chicken-breast sandwich with cheese, a chocolate bar, and two fudge-covered cookies. (I *had* to eat sweets for breakfast— doctor's orders.) For lunch I had steak with salad and fruit, and dinner was Dr. Jakubowicz's special stew. Later, if my belly growled—which wasn't often—I snacked on sliced melon or kiwi.

From my first day on the diet, I did not feel hungry, and since I'd indulged my sweet tooth in the morning, I didn't miss my nightly treats. Within five weeks, I had a natural period, my first since age 16. After six months, I was 26 pounds lighter and menstruating every four to six weeks.

Two months later, no period. I rushed out for another home-pregnancy test. *Positive!* I carried a healthy girl to term. I left the hospital at 190 pounds, and by the time my daughter was about four months old, I was down to 140. Almost three years after the birth of my daughter, my weight fluctuates between 139 and 141 pounds, and I still eat the Big Breakfast way.

So will my daughter. I want to protect her from the risky consequences of insulin resistance and diabetes. Unlike me, she will be healthy—from the start.

2

CIRCADIAN RHYTHMS 101

For our body is like a clock; if one wheel be amiss,
all the rest are disordered; the whole fabric suffers.

—*Democritus,* The Anatomy of Melancholy

It doesn't take a sleep expert to know that the presence and absence of natural light exert a powerful influence on our lives and habits. For millions of years, we've awakened to light and fallen asleep in darkness. We don't have to think about it—we naturally feel alert by day, sleepy at night. If you work a night shift, you have to fight to stay awake and struggle to sleep.

Our appetites follow this light-and-dark pattern, too. Our appetites have been hard-wired to respond to light in the early morning, when our cave-dwelling ancestors needed energy for hard work, and to diminish when the sun went down, when they needed to rest. They didn't eat after dark—they were exhausted from hunting and gathering all day, so, quite sensibly, they slept.

Fast-forward to the modern world. Electric lighting allows us to remain active—and to munch far into the night, when we used to sleep. Could it be that the obesity epidemic is somehow related to our ability to eat long after dark, when our hormonal environment doesn't support food intake and our satiety mechanisms appear to be weak? It's hard to pinpoint a single source, but it's clear that sunlight influences our body weight. The reason: circadian rhythms.

THE SKINNY

Sunlight—or the lack of it—regulates your body's circadian rhythms, which in turn govern the hormones that regulate your metabolism, hunger, mood, and cravings. If your eating patterns are out of sync with your circadian and hormonal rhythms, you'll gain weight more easily.

On the other hand, when you eat *with* your natural rhythms, your body is better able to direct the energy from the food you eat to your muscles, rather than store it as fat.

All living things—people, animals, plants, even bacteria!—experience cyclical patterns of vital processes that occur each day, in the same order. These daily rhythms, which affect our chemistry and behavior, are called *circadian,* derived from the Latin words for "approximately" (*circa*) and "day" (*dies*).

In people, circadian rhythms govern functions we don't notice: body temperature, heartbeat, and blood pressure, to name a few. They also affect how we feel: sleepy, hungry, calm, irritable. The human body repeats the cycle every 24 to 25 hours. Light stimulation (day) and the lack of it (night) keep our circadian rhythms cycling as they should.

Your "body clock" uses signals such as light and darkness to know when to release certain hormones and neurotransmitters that tell you when to wake up or go to sleep. This master clock is regulated by a part of the brain called the suprachiasmatic nucleus (SCN, see diagram at right). Located in the hypothalamus at the base of the brain, the SCN responds to light and dark. Every morning, light absorbed by the retinas of your eyes helps set the SCN. The master clock then cues

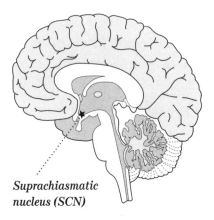

Suprachiasmatic nucleus (SCN)

other biological pacemakers, including hormone production. From the optic nerve of the eye, light travels to the SCN—a signal that it is time to be awake. It then signals to other parts of the brain to raise body temperature, produce "awake" hormones such as cortisol (see below), and stop producing melatonin, a hormone that helps bring on drowsiness and sleep produced when the retinas signal to the SCN that it is dark.

While most people associate circadian rhythms exclusively with the sleep/wake cycle, they influence much more than that. Circadian rhythms also affect our hormonal landscape, which can dramatically affect metabolism, mood, hunger, and cravings, all of which can affect our weight.

DAYLIGHT SAVING

During spring and summer, when the days are longer, you must finish eating your big breakfast before 9 A.M. and lunch before 2 P.M. During fall and winter, when hours of sunlight are reduced, you must finish eating your big breakfast by 10 A.M. and lunch before 3 P.M.

This chapter describes the ways in which those circadian rhythms affect your hormones—and your weight. The first thing you need to know is that hormones work in shifts.

HORMONES
"Day Shift" and "Night Shift"

The cycles of day and night, of sun and darkness, regulate the hormonal rhythms of the endocrine and central nervous systems. These rhythms work as a two-phase system:

1. the morning phase (day shift) that begins at dawn.
2. the night phase (night shift) that begins at sunset.

On each shift, hormones that regulate metabolism, energy levels, appetite, and mood change by the hour. Let's look at a few of the hormones that play a significant role in body weight.

DAY SHIFT *(DAWN)*:

▶ **ADRENALINE** This hormone promotes wakefulness, alertness, mental concentration, and problem-solving ability. It also promotes *thermogenesis,* the production of heat by metabolic processes. Thermogenesis burns body fat.

▶ **CORTISOL** This hormone converts protein into muscle and energy and contributes to maintaining the levels of glucose for many hours. It also regulates the body's "emergency system" that guarantees minimal levels of glucose in the blood to fuel the brain.

▶ **SEROTONIN** You'll learn more about this hormonelike brain chemical on page 35. For now, it's enough to know that it's crucial to maintain optimum serotonin levels to regulate mood and control carbohydrate cravings.

▶ **INSULIN SENSITIVITY** Insulin is the hormone that takes energy (glucose) from the food we eat out of the bloodstream and into the muscles, so they can use it for fuel. This means that the body is better able to use carbohydrates for energy.

NIGHT SHIFT *(SUNSET)*:

▶ **HUMAN GROWTH HORMONE (HGH)** This hormone helps the body utilize fat reserves as fuel, thereby burning fat that leads to weight loss. It begins its ascent at sunset and reaches its highest level around midnight.

▶ **SEROTONIN** Along with melatonin, serotonin begins a gradual, steady increase beginning in the early evening, to get us ready for sleep. (This is often when food cravings are highest.)

▶ **INSULIN SENSITIVITY** Insulin's ability to get glucose out of the blood and into the muscles diminishes as the day wears on. This means that eating sweets and starches at night will most likely result in storing their energy as body fat.

Eating in Time

Your body can use the food you eat to provide energy and build muscle—or store fat. Fortunately, you have some say in the matter. It's as simple as knowing how types of food affect your metabolic and hormonal environment at the time you consume them.

DAY-SHIFT METABOLISM

CORTISOL RULES MORNING METABOLISM. This hormone helps convert protein to energy. Eaten in the morning, high-protein foods such as cheese, milk, and eggs undergo changes that better preserve and build muscle mass, provide energy, increase alertness and mental concentration, and keep blood glucose levels steady for many hours. Steady glucose levels keep hunger at bay.

One more thing: The complicated chemical reactions that occur when you eat protein in the morning, rather than at night, raise body temperature and dramatically accelerate metabolism. This makes it easier not to gain weight during the rest of the day, even if you eat a lot.

IF IT'S MORNING, IT'S TIME FOR CARBS. As you now know, the body is more sensitive to the action of insulin in the morning. When you eat starches in the morning, the slight rise in insulin introduces the sugar into the muscles, increasing energy rather than fat reserves. Translation: Eaten in the morning, when insulin is most efficient, sweets and starches won't cause weight gain.

Consuming carbohydrates in the morning also maintains the levels of serotonin throughout the day, decreasing the addiction to sweets that overweight people typically battle in the afternoon.

NIGHT-SHIFT METABOLISM

PROTEIN, FRUITS, AND VEGGIES RULE. I promised that my plan would allow you to eat all the foods you love, and you can—just not at night, because eating carbohydrates at night is a recipe for weight gain. This hard fact has everything to do with the action of insulin, or rather, the *inaction* of insulin.

At night, your body is less responsive to insulin. So it's best for your health and weight *not* to eat those foods that we know cause a large, sustained release of insulin. Generally speaking, those foods include all your favorites, from mac and cheese to chocolate cake. If you eat starch and sugar, your insulin levels will skyrocket and stay high for a long time.

This sustained elevation of insulin is not good for your body. It raises triglycerides, reduces "good" HDL cholesterol, raises blood pressure, and promotes atherosclerosis; it doesn't help your weight, either. That starchy meal or triple-layer cake causes

HOW OUR BODY CLOCK AFFECTS
OUR BODY FAT

I've thrown a lot of science at you. Perhaps you're thinking, Enough of the theory. What actually happens when I eat out of sync? What does my brain do? How are my hormones affected? What's the effect on my body?

Here's a sample day of eating out of sync, from sunrise to sunset—and beyond. It's not pretty.

▶ **6:30 A.M.:** You skip breakfast. The brain activates its emergency systems. Powered by cortisol, your body cannibalizes proteins from your muscles and skin. Continue to skip breakfast and your body will eventually carry more fat than muscle, which slows your metabolism and makes weight gain more likely. Skipping breakfast also deprives your brain of the serotonin it needs to fight off midafternoon carb cravings—so don't be surprised if you find yourself at the vending machine, desperate for a sugar fix.

▶ **NOON:** You're starving (you skipped breakfast, remember?) so you plow into a burger and fries or a few slices of pizza. At this time of day your sensitivity to insulin is already less than optimal. So the

insulin to work overtime. Because this hormone is not very effective at transporting glucose to your muscles, it directs it to your fat reserves. You heard me right. Eating sweets and starches at night actually encourages your body to store fat while you sleep.

Skipping Breakfast
Puts the Brain on High Alert

The brain's only source of fuel is glucose. To get glucose, you need to eat, and you particularly need to eat breakfast, because glucose from your high-carbohydrate, lower-protein meal will circulate in your bloodstream rather than go where it's needed—your muscles. Eventually, this excess glucose will be stored as body fat.

▶ **3:00–4:00 P.M.:** You're at your desk, feeling tired and irritable. That's because, having skipped breakfast, your brain is now crying out for something sweet to calm the irritability caused by low levels of serotonin. Desperate to feel better, you reach for a chocolate bar to restore energy and mood. If you do this daily, your brain and body associate sweets and starches with feeling good. You may be caught in a cycle of addiction, and it must be broken.

▶ **6:00 P.M.:** You're frustrated and upset at having overeaten today— again. You figure you've blown it today; you might as well blow it tonight, too. So you eat what you want for dinner—typically, another high-carbohydrate meal. By now, insulin is even less efficient than it was at lunchtime, so most of those calories will be stored as body fat.

▶ **MIDNIGHT AND BEYOND:** Unable to sleep, you dish out a bowl of ice cream, nibble chips, or pop chocolate kisses, derailing the ability of HGH to use fat reserves as fuel. Plus, eating now ensures that you won't be hungry for breakfast—which means the destructive cycle begins anew when you wake up.

it's the first meal after an eight-hour fast. (That's where the word *breakfast* comes from; you're breaking your nightly fast.) Breakfast is the most widely skipped meal of the day—and your brain really, really doesn't like it when you skip breakfast.

Fortunately, the brain has emergency systems to ensure that it gets the glucose it needs. These systems have but one goal: to maintain stable levels of glucose in the blood. Activation of the system depends on the time of day that low glucose levels occur, since the brain and body react very differently to skipping breakfast than to not eating at night.

THE MORNING EMERGENCY SYSTEM

When you don't eat when you wake up, thereby extending your nocturnal fast, your brain goes into emergency mode. The action of cortisol in the emergency mode stimulates the destruction of muscle protein and its conversion into glucose in order to maintain the levels of blood glucose until the fast is broken.

When you first wake up in the morning, your brain has a 15-minute "reserve" of blood sugar (glucose) before levels begin to fall. This descent in blood sugar activates Emergency System Phase 1: The liver releases its own reserve of sugar. This reserve maintains the levels of glucose in the blood for another 15 minutes. The clock continues to tick. If, by the time the liver's reserve is exhausted, you still haven't broken your fast, the brain understands this scarcity as an unending famine: It believes food will never arrive.

This causes your brain to activate Emergency System Phase 2: It signals the release of cortisol, which produces a massive destruction of the proteins in your skin and muscle. The proteins in these tissues are converted to amino acids, which leave the muscle and enter your liver, where they are converted to glucose.

You might ask: Why can't body fat be converted to glucose? Because in the morning, the hormone in control is cortisol, and it uses protein as reserve fuel. The hormone that burns fat as reserve fuel, HGH, is active at night.

The result: Skip breakfast and your body's "day shift" hormones ensure that you'll burn muscle, not fat.

You'll also be slightly ditzy—mentally foggy and fatigued. The highs and lows of glucose produced by a deficient breakfast put the brain at a disadvantage. When you skip breakfast, 80 percent of your brain must be engaged in activating its emergency systems. That unfortunately leaves only 20 percent for mental processes such as problem solving and learning, which you typically need at work. A full breakfast is essential to keeping your mind alert—and no, a large cup of coffee doesn't count.

THE EVENING EMERGENCY SYSTEM

Your brain needs glucose 24 hours a day, even when you sleep. When we sleep, we don't eat. How can the brain get the glucose it needs? That's where HGH comes in. It burns fat reserves as fuel. Not many of my patients have a problem with that! On the other hand, if you eat carbohydrates at dinner or beyond, HGH's ability to mobilize fat reserves diminishes.

Serotonin and the Chemistry of Craving

The rise and fall of serotonin determines when you get sleepy, when you wake up, and when (and what) you eat. It also has a profound effect on mood. Put all these qualities together and you can see why it's crucial to get serotonin production in sync. Do that and you avoid the midafternoon crash and master your carb cravings.

Manufactured by the brain, serotonin is a neurotransmitter, a type of chemical that helps relay signals from one area of the brain to another. Most of our brain cells—all 40 million or so—are influenced by serotonin, including those related to mood, sleep, and appetite.

Here's a snapshot of serotonin's "schedule." It rises at dusk and stays up most of the night. As serotonin rises, and levels of stimulant hormones fall, you get sleepy. At dawn, the gradual increase of daylight stimulates the pineal gland, and it stops secreting serotonin. The cycle begins anew as daylight fades and darkness falls.

TO LOSE WEIGHT, TURN IN BEFORE MIDNIGHT

As day turns into night, your body's release of growth hormone (HGH) climbs. This hormone reaches its peak between midnight and 1 A.M., and it is during this period that HGH is most efficient at burning body fat as reserve fuel.

If you typically get to bed before 12 A.M., you're getting the maximum benefit from HGH. But if your normal bedtime is after midnight, you're missing out. Studies show that the HGH levels of people who go to bed after midnight are lower than those of people who turn in earlier.

When your serotonin levels are optimal, you think better, sleep better, and feel better. You have fewer cravings and weight loss comes more easily. But when levels drop too low, you feel depressed and irritable, may crave sweets and starches, and are more likely to overeat.

Overweight people's ebbs and flows of serotonin are more extreme. First, they tend to have higher-than-typical levels in the morning, which curtails hunger and cravings. Result: They skip breakfast. By midafternoon (around 3:00 or 4:00 P.M.) their serotonin levels plummet—especially if they're on a low-carbohydrate diet and have also skipped breakfast. This serotonin "low" leaves them tired and irritable. They also crave something sweet. They may not know that carbohydrates, which raise serotonin levels naturally, act like a natural tranquilizer, but their bodies do.

But there's more to the story. The serotonin low also involves insulin, as well as the amino acid tryptophan, which the brain

The Big Breakfast Diet program is designed to help you get maximum benefit from the nighttime release of HGH. The key points for nighttime eating are:

▶ Get to sleep well before midnight.
▶ Eat your last meal of the day at least three hours before turning in.
▶ No sweets or starches after breakfast—stick to lean protein and low-sugar fruits and veggies.
▶ If you must snack at night, stick to a cup or bowl of The Stew (page 52) or any of the "Free Foods" listed on page 65.
▶ Avoid HGH pills or potions. Although studies show that HGH increases muscle mass and decreases body fat, HGH supplements sold online or over the counter are unproven, ineffective, and possibly dangerous.

uses to make serotonin. Although amino acids come from protein foods, *carbs alone* determine whether enough tryptophan makes it into your brain.

When you eat sweets and starches, your insulin levels rise. Insulin directs many amino acids into cells throughout the body. That suppresses blood levels of the amino acids that compete with tryptophan for entrance into the brain. Carbs send these "competitor" amino acids elsewhere, allowing tryptophan to enter the brain to be converted to serotonin.

However, the exaggerated elevation of insulin that overweight people produce when they consume sweets and starches (that's insulin resistance, remember?) causes a greater increase in serotonin and a "feel-good" effect. This perpetuates the addiction to sweets and starches that many overweight people experience.

Fortunately, there's a simple solution: Get your sweets and starches in the morning! This will ensure that your brain has the serotonin it needs to keep your carb cravings in check.

THE
PLAN

3

THE BIG BREAKFAST DIET:
TWO SIMPLE RULES FOR SUCCESS

ow that you understand the science behind my weight-loss plan, you're ready to turn theory into action. This chapter spells out the basics—everything you need to know to make the Big Breakfast Diet the last weight-loss plan you'll ever need.

After you digest my two simple guidelines (I've dubbed them the Big Breakfast Two), familiarize yourself with the Servings List and the Fruit and Vegetable Lists at the end of the chapter—as well as the formulas you plug them into in chapters 4 and 5. These are the cornerstones of my plan. The meal plans found in chapter 6 are built from them, and once you've internalized them, you can use them to design your own tasty meals. (No need to memorize these lists. Simply photocopy two sets: one for your fridge, another for your wallet.)

A word about calories: Don't give them another thought. The women in my study consumed about 600 calories for breakfast, and another 600 calories split between lunch and dinner. That's not a huge amount; in fact, it's the minimum number of calories recommended per day. However, if you've been starving yourself on 1,000 calories a day or less on other diets, 1,200 calories is a vast improvement. Before they came to me, some of my patients existed on 800 or even 500 calories a day—not only misguided, but dangerous—and were still gaining weight.

That said, it's possible to bump your daily calories to

THE SKINNY

Follow my two simple rules for success—a.k.a. the Big Breakfast Two—on the following pages and you can't go wrong. And stick close to the Formulas (page 172) and the Servings List (page 54), the cornerstone of my plan, which you can use to "build" your meals. The Fruit and Vegetable Lists rank fruits and veggies according to sugar content per serving, to build your lunch and dinner. (*Hint:* The less sugar they contain, the more of them you can eat.) If you're a vegetarian, adapt the program to your needs using the guidelines on page 48.

3,000 (women) or 3,200 (men) and still lose weight—*if* you eat in sync. Begin the plan with the recommended seven servings of protein at breakfast, but if you find that you're hungry at night, increase your servings of morning protein, one serving at a time, until your hunger subsides. (Don't worry about calories. They don't count on this plan, remember? Simply increase your protein servings in the morning until you no longer get hungry at night.) Remember: Protein, especially when consumed at breakfast, has a high satiety factor. As a bonus, protein in the morning gets your metabolism into high gear.

Without further ado, here are the Big Breakfast Two. The more diligent you are in following them, the more weight you can potentially lose.

RULE #1
Always eat breakfast. Always.

Whether you wake up at 6:30 or 8:00 in the morning, start eating breakfast within 15 minutes of rolling out of bed. You can down your entire breakfast, if you like, or just a small portion of it to get things started. This gives your brain the glucose it needs to function after eight or so hours without food, and it prevents the activation of your body's morning emergency system.

Breakfast is the weight-loss "gift" that keeps on giving. First, a morning meal shifts your body from an energy-conserving state to calorie-burning. Second, research shows that those who eat breakfast concentrate better and are more productive than those who skip it. Plus, need I remind you—if you skip it, you're more likely to overeat later on because you're ravenously hungry.

If you're not used to eating in the morning, I sympathize. Many of my patients had skipped breakfast for years, which is part of the reason they'd gotten heavy in the first place. But if you make the effort to fit this meal into your life, you'll see—and feel—the rewards.

If you skip breakfast because you are in a rush, you need to make the time to eat. If you skip it because you're simply not hungry in the morning, well, fake it. In chapter 4, you'll learn how to retrain your body to experience hunger when it's most advantageous to eat.

For those of you who say you are not hungry in the morning, try making yourself eat breakfast around the same time every day for two weeks (if it's still hard, try eating your breakfast in shifts over the course of an hour). After two weeks, you'll get used to eating at that time and your body will begin to expect breakfast when you first wake up.

You don't have to scarf down your entire morning meal within 15 minutes, either. As mentioned, it's perfectly fine to eat it "in shifts," as long as you finish before 9 A.M. (10 A.M. in fall and winter).

RULE #2
Eat in Sync. Always.

For my plan to work for you, it's critical that you honor both your day-shift and night-shift metabolisms. In a nutshell, this means:

▶ Bring on the protein!

▶ Sweets and starches by 9 A.M. (or by 10 A.M. in fall and winter)

▶ Lunch by 2 P.M. (or by 3 P.M. in fall and winter)

At breakfast and lunch you *must* adhere to the recommended serving sizes of proteins, fats, and carbohydrates. Each meal contains the optimum portions of satisfying protein, healthy fats, and energizing carbohydrates to satisfy your hunger, accelerate your metabolism, and discourage cravings.

YOU MUST *CONSUME AT LEAST 7 SERVINGS OF PROTEIN AT BREAKFAST.* Eaten in the morning, high-protein foods undergo changes that help preserve and build muscle, sharpen your mind, and keep hunger at bay for hours. Further, the chemical reactions that occur when you eat protein in the A.M. raise your body temperature and dramatically accelerate metabolism. Research shows that protein can increase postmeal calorie burn by as much as 35 percent!

SWEETS AND STARCHES IN THE MORNING. Because insulin is more efficient in the morning, it's better at introducing glucose into the muscles (rather than diverting them to body-fat reserves).

Your breakfast sweets and starches will also help manufacture serotonin, which will help break the addiction to sweets that many overweight people battle in the midafternoon.

LUNCH BEFORE 2 P.M./3 P.M. As afternoon passes into evening, the hormones that transform food into body fat rise, promoting weight gain. This means you want to cool it on the sweets and starches and load up on protein, veggies, and fruit. The proteins help extend the hunger-reducing effect of breakfast. You'll select fruits and veggies according to their sugar content—you can eat more of the ones that contain less sugar (Veggie and Fruit Groups A), and eat fewer of the ones that are higher in sugar (Veggie Group B and Fruit Groups B–D).

I'm willing to bet that you won't be hungry for lunch, at least at first. But don't skip this meal, even if you're still full from breakfast. Think of it this way: Eat now, when you're not hungry,

THE 9 A.M. RULE

I've explained that to eat in sync, you must finish your morning meal before 9 A.M. (see box on page 28 for Daylight Saving). But what happens if you get up and eat very early—say, at 5 A.M.? Or, alternatively, if you sleep in on a Saturday or Sunday morning, or work the night shift, and miss your 9 A.M. breakfast "deadline"?

Let's tackle sleeping late first. Sleeping in after a long night is part of life. The solution: Eat immediately after you wake up. If you "wait for lunch," your body is in a fasting state. This means your body will "steal" proteins from your muscles and—to protect you from starving—store the rest as abdominal fat.

or risk eating later, when cravings are raging and you may not be able to manage your appetite.

IN THE AFTERNOON AND EVENING, PROTEIN, FRUITS, AND VEGGIES RULE. By now, you know that evening carbs interfere with the release of growth hormone and promote fat storage while you sleep. This hard fact has everything to do with the actions of insulin. Or rather, its *inaction.* So enjoy pizza, pasta, bread, or bakery items in the morning, when your body can best utilize them.

In the first few days of the program, you may feel a bit hungry as your body gets accustomed to eating in sync. To quiet lingering hunger pangs at any time of day (or night!), spoon out a bowl of The Stew (page 52). You can also opt for a half cup of reduced-fat cottage cheese (mixed with Splenda and cinnamon, if you like) or up to 3 servings of low-fat cheese or lean meat, fish, or poultry.

Also, no matter how late you get up, eat lunch before 2 P.M., even if you've just eaten breakfast and are not hungry. Your hormonal landscape hasn't changed, even if your personal schedule is off, and you must eat according to your hormonal rhythms.

What if you rise at 5 A.M. and finish breakfast soon after? Well, I'd bet that you feel full after only a few bites. That's because your satiety hormones are very strong early in the morning. The only problem is, most people who eat a tiny breakfast so early want to eat everything in sight come late afternoon. Solution: Eat your regular 5 A.M. breakfast, then add one or two more "breakfasts" at 7 or 8 A.M. (How does a slice of cake and a glass of milk and a smoothie or shake sound?) Make sure you eat all your protein servings, too, to accelerate your metabolism and avoid hunger all day long.

TAKE ADVANTAGE OF THE BIG BREAKFAST SHAKE, SMOOTHIE, AND STEW.
All three "S" recipes (starting on page 50) are integral to the
Big Breakfast Diet. The Shake and The Smoothie are packed
with good proteins for breakfast—and there's a bonus. As you'll
learn in the next chapter, you *must* drink at least two glasses of
milk, preferably nonfat, as part of your morning meal. A shake or
smoothie is a quick, tasty way to consume one or both servings.

The Stew is low-sugar but full of fuel to carry you throughout
the day.

PICK YOUR PLAN:
Relaxed or Turbocharged

My plan can be a challenge, at least at first. Not because you'll be
hungry—as long as you eat enough proteins, you won't be—but
because my plan flies in the face of the typical Western way of
eating.

When you eat out of sync, as most overweight people do,
you consume most of your calories after 5 P.M. On my plan, you
consume most of your calories before 9 A.M.—a daunting task
when you're used to eating out of sync.

There are two ways you can follow the plan (think of it as a
"choose your own adventure"). Pick the speed that suits you.

PLAN A: TURBOCHARGED With this option, you follow the diet
exactly as the Big Breakfast study participants did. That means
you will consume 610 to 850 calories at breakfast, and primarily
vegetables and fruits with some protein for lunch and little or no
dinner. (To see what my Big Breakfast Group ate, see the chart on
page 5.) No carbs at lunch or dinner unless they're in fruits and
veggies. No fats or other oils. Period. Your reward: You'll lose
weight fast.

If you're full after breakfast and lunch—and you should be—you can kick it up a notch and skip dinner altogether. If you go to sleep without dinner, your body will burn fat to use as energy. Skipping dinner (though not always socially feasible) also has the benefit of making you wake up feeling very hungry, which will help you eat a big breakfast.

PLAN B: RELAXED This option may be a slightly more realistic way to incorporate this way of eating into your lifestyle—at least at first. You may consume more calories, even at breakfast, than the study participants. In fact, you may consume upward of 3,000 calories at breakfast. That's fine. I've prescribed this version of the diet to the patients in my practice for years. You see, the success of my plan is not based on calories, but on *types of foods and when you eat them,* and the effect of certain foods on the body's hormonal environment. Eating too much breakfast is simply not possible as long as you follow the formula and finish breakfast before 9 A.M. (10 A.M. during fall and winter).

On the Relaxed plan, you may also include small amounts of fats in your lunch and dinner options—a tablespoon or two of oil on your salads, a bit of mayonnaise, some butter, or other "fat-y" ingredients. The addition of these ingredients simply makes lunch and dinner more palatable. You may not lose weight as quickly, but you *will* lose it. If you become discouraged that you're not losing weight as quickly as hoped, crank up to the Turbocharged plan.

Sometimes it's preferable to reduce the speed of weight loss in order to feel comfortable with the diet. But remember, never eat starches at night. If you go to a social gathering, there are ways to keep to your diet. At a barbecue, eat the meat and the salad, but not the potato, the bread, or the rice. If you are offered a sandwich or a pizza, don't eat the bread, eat only the protein. All this will now be possible because you will have control over your cravings. And you can always save your favorite foods for breakfast.

I recommend that you follow the Turbocharged option first. It's the plan with documented success, and as a scientist, I believe in reproducible results. That said, if you don't think you can follow this plan's stringent parameters, try Plan B first. If you don't lose weight at the pace you're expecting, switch to the Turbocharged option—and watch the pounds slip away.

The Vegetarian Option

Can you follow the Big Breakfast Diet plan if you're a vegetarian? You bet. Whether you're a lacto-ovo vegetarian who consumes milk and egg products, a lacto vegetarian who consumes milk products but no eggs, or a vegan who avoids all animal products, you'll simply rely on plant-based sources of protein to meet your protein needs.

If you're a lacto- or lacto-ovo vegetarian, you'll find it easy to get the plan's recommended protein servings. Sources of protein include: low-fat or fat-free milk, yogurt, cheese, and cottage cheese; eggs; tofu, tempeh, and meat analogues made with soy; legumes, seeds, nuts and nut butters; and grains. To get your seven servings of protein at breakfast, for example, you might enjoy a bean and cheese burrito or a veggie burger, or whip up a tofu scramble or shake. I also recommend doubling the servings of whey (to 6 tablespoons) when you prepare The Shake or The Smoothie. If you also eat fish, the plan becomes easier still—fish is an amazing source of lean protein, as long as it's prepared without breading or fat. (For vegetarian-friendly menus and recipes, see page 130.) Finally, a diet consisting primarily of vegetables (made up of amino acid chains) won't satiate hunger as easily. Therefore, vegetarians are encouraged to double up on many of their vegetable servings at breakfast and lunch, and to particularly note the snacking list on page 95 for in-between meals. If you're a vegan, you need to be mindful of getting enough of the nutrients listed below. The foods suggested count toward either your protein (P) or carbohydrate (C) servings.

VITAMIN B12: fortified soy products and beverages (P) and fortified cereals (C).

VITAMIN D: fortified soy beverages (P) and sunshine (your skin makes vitamin D when it's exposed to a safe amount of sun each day).

CALCIUM: tofu (if made with calcium sulfate) (P), soy-based beverage with added calcium (P), breakfast cereal with added calcium (C), fruit juice with added calcium (C), collards, turnip greens, and other dark-green leafy vegetables (C). (Note: To get enough calcium from green leafies, you'll have to consume a lot of them.)

IRON: ready-to-eat cereals with added iron (C), spinach (C), beans (kidney, pinto) (P), peas (black-eyed) (P), lentils (P), enriched and whole-grain breads (C). To help your body absorb nonanimal sources of iron, eat foods rich in vitamin C—such as strawberries, citrus fruits, tomatoes, cabbage, and broccoli—at the same time you eat iron-rich foods.

ZINC: whole grains (especially the germ and bran) (C), whole-wheat bread (C), legumes, nuts, and tofu (P).

One more thing: If you don't eat any animal products, ask your doctor if you should take a vitamin-mineral supplement to ensure that you get all the nutrients your body needs.

THE BIG 3:
RECIPES

Tasty, quick, and convenient, The Shake, The Smoothie, and The Stew are vital parts of the Big Breakfast plan. So drag out your blender and slow cooker—you'll need them!

The delicious Shake and Smoothie contain milk, soy milk, or yogurt, along with whey protein; in the morning all are excellent sources of high-quality proteins that accelerate metabolism and control hunger. The Shake or The Smoothie provide a quick, tasty way to consume two servings of milk at breakfast. Of course, you can always simply drink 16 ounces of low-fat milk with your meal. The low-sugar, slow-release carbohydrates in The Stew give you the fuel your body needs at precisely the right time of day. Most important, all three recipes are easy to prepare.

✳ The Shake

When it comes to The Shake, use your creativity. There are any number of flavorings you can add. For example, try a Shake made with chocolate protein powder and a tablespoon of peanut butter, or make a piña colada Shake with vanilla protein powder, coconut flavoring, and a quarter cup of pineapple. Experiment to find the perfect flavor and don't forget to write it down so you can replicate it.

Makes 1 portion

1 cup (8 ounces) low-fat milk or soy milk

3 tablespoons sugar-free whey protein powder, any flavor

A few drops of flavoring extract, such as vanilla, orange, banana, or coconut, or 1½ teaspoons peanut butter or almond butter

A dash of spice: ground cinnamon, nutmeg, or ginger

2 to 4 ice cubes (optional)

Splenda or other sugar substitute (see Note)

Place the milk, protein powder, and flavoring and/or spice of your choice in a blender, adding ice cubes, if desired, and blend on low speed until The Shake is smooth and creamy. Add sugar substitute to taste.

NOTE: Do not use sugar instead of the artificial sweetener; regular sugar has a negative impact on insulin and blood glucose levels.

THIS WHEY OR
THAT WHEY?

There are many whey protein products on the market. Commercially, whey is often mixed with other ingredients and may contain lactose, fat, and minerals. Whey protein isolate is the purest form; it contains between 90 and 95 percent protein and little, if any, fat or lactose. Whey protein concentrate, a protein powder supplement with 80 percent protein content, is the most commonly available form—3 tablespoons contain about 16 grams of protein, which is perfect for mixing into The Shake or The Smoothie. (If you are allergic to or have an aversion to milk, yogurt, or soy, substitute 3 tablespoons of whey for the serving and mix it with water and fruit for a smoothie.) Note: Whey should only be used to supplement a meal and increase satiety.

3 TABLESPOONS OF WHEY PROTEIN POWDER = 1 MILK PROTEIN SERVING

✳ The Smoothie

Filled with protein, this smoothie will start you off on the right track. Use any fruit you like from Fruit Groups A, B, C, or D (page 67), regardless of its sugar content, to flavor your breakfast Smoothie. Make it first thing in the morning and start slurping it down immediately to kickstart your Big Breakfast.

Makes 1 portion

> 1 cup (8 ounces) plain low-fat yogurt
> 3 tablespoons sugar-free plain whey protein powder
> 1 cup chopped fresh fruit,
>   or 1 cup partially thawed frozen fruit
> Splenda or other sugar substitute (see Note)

Place the yogurt, protein powder, and fruit in a blender and blend on low speed, increasing the speed to high, until the smoothie is smooth and creamy. Add sugar substitute to taste.

NOTE: Do not use sugar instead of the artificial sweetener; regular sugar has a negative impact on insulin and blood glucose levels.

✳ The Stew

This tasty, hearty veggie stew is so easy to prepare—just dump the ingredients in your Crock-Pot, set it to low, and go. When you come home from work, you'll have a delicious, flavorful dish that's brimming with hunger-curbing fiber and plant nutrients that help protect against a wide variety of diseases, including heart disease and diabetes. If you're hungry after dinner, or between meals, you can ladle up a bowl of stew, guilt-free. A pot of stew can last several days or more, depending on how often you eat it. But don't be surprised if you're cooking up a pot twice a week (it can simmer in the Crock-Pot while you're at work). Enjoy a bowl between meals, too—it's that good!

Makes 4 to 6 portions

4 cups vegetable broth (preferably low-sodium)
3 cups water
5 large tomatoes, chopped,
  or 1 can (14.5 ounces) diced tomatoes
3 bell peppers, any color, seeded and chopped
2 medium-size zucchini, chopped
2 cups chopped green or red cabbage
2 cups broccoli or cauliflower florets,
  or 1 cup each of both
1 medium-size eggplant, chopped
1 cup chopped onion
½ pound mushrooms, any variety, trimmed and chopped
1 cup string beans, cut in half crosswise
1 cup chopped carrots
1 can (14 ounces) artichoke hearts packed in water,
  drained and quartered
1½ teaspoons dried oregano
1 handful fresh basil and parsley leaves,
  or 1 teaspoon dried basil and 1 teaspoon dried parsley
1 to 3 whole cloves garlic, peeled
Salt and freshly ground black pepper
Crushed red pepper flakes

Place the vegetable broth, water, tomatoes, bell peppers, zucchini, cabbage, broccoli and/or cauliflower, eggplant, onion, mushrooms, string beans, carrots, artichoke hearts, oregano, basil and parsley, and garlic in a Crock-Pot and stir well. Season the mixture with salt, black pepper, and red pepper flakes to taste. Cook the stew on low heat until the flavors develop, 7 to 9 hours. Before serving, taste the stew for seasoning, adding more salt and/or black pepper as necessary.

THE BIG BREAKFAST DIET

SERVINGS LIST

Following the principles of the Food Exchanges list used by the American Diabetes Association, the list you'll find here is the cornerstone of the Big Breakfast Diet plan, the one tool you need to design your meals. I used the list to create the thirty tasty breakfasts, lunches, and dinners you'll find in chapter 6. But once you're familiar with the list, you can design your own meals— the creative possibilities are endless.

Dairy

Milk or yogurt, whether dairy or soy, are absolutely key to kicking off your big breakfast proteins.

MILK

	ONE SERVING EQUALS
Milk, whole, 2%, or 1%	1 cup (8 ounces)
Milk, powdered fat-free	⅓ cup plus water
Hot chocolate mix, sugar-free	3 teaspoons plus water
Buttermilk, low-fat or fat-free	1 cup (8 ounces)
Evaporated milk, whole or skim	½ cup (4 ounces)
Soy milk	1 cup (8 ounces)
Yogurt, plain low-fat	¾ cup (6 ounces)
Yogurt, artificially sweetened fat-free	¾ cup (6 ounces)
Yogurt, plain fat-free	¾ cup (6 ounces)
Whipped topping, low-fat or fat-free	2 tablespoons

CHEESE

	ONE SERVING EQUALS
Cottage cheese, regular, low-fat, or fat-free	¼ cup (2 ounces)

American, Cheddar, Monterey Jack, Swiss, feta, mozzarella, regular or fat-free	Two slices (1 ounce)
Parmesan or Romano, grated	2 tablespoons
Ricotta	¼ cup (2 ounces)

EGGS

	ONE SERVING EQUALS
Whole eggs	One egg (no more than three eggs per week)
Egg whites	Three egg whites
Egg substitute	¼ cup

Meat, Poultry, and Fish

Load up on your animal-based proteins early in the day.

MEAT

	ONE SERVING EQUALS
Beef, trimmed lean cuts *Steaks, including T-bone, porterhouse, and flank and top round steaks; roasts including rib, chuck, and rump; and sirloin or tenderloin*	1 ounce
Beef, cuts with some fat marbling *Including ground beef, corned beef, short ribs, and meat loaf*	1 ounce
Veal *Roast, lean chops, or cutlet*	1 ounce
Pork *Tenderloin, chops, fresh ham, spareribs, and ground pork*	1 ounce
Bacon	1 ounce (three slices; also counts as three servings of fat)
Canadian bacon	1 ounce (one slice)
Lamb *Roast, lean chops, or ground lamb*	1 ounce

Lean cold cuts
Including roast beef, ham, bologna,
pastrami, turkey, and chicken   1 ounce (two slices)

Salami or pepperoni   1 ounce

Hot dogs   One small hot dog

Sausages
Including Italian sausage,
Polish sausage, bratwurst, and
kielbasa (beef, turkey, or chicken)   1 ounce

Breakfast sausage   1 ounce

Meatballs   Three medium-size
                                           meatballs

POULTRY   ONE SERVING EQUALS

Chicken or turkey,
white meat (no skin)   1 ounce

Chicken or turkey,
dark meat (no skin)   1 ounce

Chicken or turkey, ground   1 ounce

Other poultry
Including Cornish hen, duck, pheasant,
and goose (no skin)   1 ounce

SEAFOOD   ONE SERVING EQUALS

Fish, fresh or frozen
Including salmon, swordfish,
flounder, sole, and tuna   1 ounce

Fish, canned in water
Including tuna, salmon, and mackerel   1 drained ounce

Herring, smoked (no cream)   1 ounce

Salmon, smoked   1 ounce

Sardines, canned   Two medium-size sardines

Fresh shellfish
Crab, lobster, shrimp, clams,
oysters, mussels, or scallops   1 ounce

Beans, Legumes, and Soy Foods

The foods on this list are high in carbohydrates and should therefore only be eaten in the morning.

	ONE SERVING EQUALS
Tofu	½ cup (4 ounces)
Tempeh	¼ cup (2 ounces)
Tempeh bacon	3 slices (2 ounces)
Meat analogs *Including veggie sausage or burger and textured vegetable protein*	1 ounce
Legumes *Including dried beans, chickpeas (garbanzo beans), peas, and lentils*	½ cup cooked
Lima beans	⅔ cup cooked
Hummus	2 tablespoons

Breads, Crackers, Grains, and Pastas

Help yourself to these carbohydrates at breakfast *only*.

BREADS AND CRACKERS	ONE SERVING EQUALS
Sandwich bread *Including White, whole wheat, whole grain, rye, or pumpernickel*	One slice ⅜ to ½ inch thick
Bread, "light" or reduced-calorie	Two slices
French or Italian bread	One slice ½ inch thick
Dinner roll	One small roll
Biscuit	One small biscuit
Croissant	One croissant about 3 by 2 inches
Bagel	One half of a small bagel (1 ounce)

English muffin	One half of an English muffin (1 ounce)
Hamburger or hot dog bun	One half of a hamburger or hot dog bun from a package (1 ounce)
Pita	One half of a 6-inch pita
Tortilla, white or whole wheat	One half of an 8-inch tortilla
Taco shells or corn tortillas	Two 6-inch taco shells or tortillas
Corn bread or corn muffin	A 2-inch square piece or 1 muffin
Bread sticks	Four bread sticks 4 inches long, ½ inch in diameter
Croutons	¾ cup
Bread crumbs, dry	3 tablespoons

CRACKERS AND SNACK FOODS

ONE SERVING EQUALS

Soda crackers	Six 2 by 2–inch crackers
Oyster crackers	24 crackers
Whole-wheat crackers	Five 2 by 2–inch crackers
Rye crispbread	Two pieces
Rice crackers	20 rice crackers
Rice cakes or popcorn cakes	Two 4-inch cakes or 5 mini cakes
Melba toast	Four slices
Matzo	One 5 by 5–inch piece
Pretzels, salted hard	1 ounce
Chips, tortilla or potato (fat free or baked)	15 to 20 chips
Chips, pita	14 chips

Popcorn, low-fat microwave	3 cups popped
Popcorn, air-popped (no fat added)	3 cups popped

CEREAL

ONE SERVING EQUALS

Puffed grains, unfrosted *Including puffed wheat, barley, and rice*	1½ cups
Shredded wheat	1 large biscuit or ½ cup spoon-size biscuits
Unsweetened cereal, ready-to-eat *Including cornflakes, Rice Crispies, and Breakfast "Os"*	¾ cup
Bran cereal	½ cup
Sugar-frosted cereal	½ cup
Granola, low-fat	¼ cup
Grape-Nuts and müesli	¼ cup
Hot cereal, unsweetened *Including oatmeal and cream of wheat*	½ cup cooked
Grits	½ cup cooked
Wheat germ	3 tablespoons

PASTAS, RICE, AND OTHER GRAINS

ONE SERVING EQUALS

Noodles *Including egg noodles, soba noodles, and udon noodles*	1 cup cooked
Pasta, unfilled *Including spaghetti, macaroni, and penne*	⅓ cup cooked
Pasta, filled *Including ravioli and tortellini*	4 to 5 cooked
Chow mein noodles	½ cup
Rice, white or brown	⅓ cup cooked
Barley, bulgar, millet, and quinoa	½ cup cooked
Couscous	⅓ cup cooked

PREPARED AND FAST FOODS

Here is a just a sampling of some prepared and fast foods you might come across and how you can incorporate them into your Big Breakfast formula (page 75).

MEAL	ONE SERVING EQUALS	ONE SERVING COUNTS FOR
Bean-style soup	1 cup (8 ounces)	1 protein 1 carbohydrate
Broth-based soup *Including vegetable beef and chicken noodle*	1 cup (8 ounces)	1 carbohydrate
Burrito, beef	One burrito (5 to 7 ounces)	1 protein 3 carbohydrate 1 fat
Chicken breast or wing, breaded or fried	One piece	4 protein 1 carbohydrate 2 fat
Chicken nuggets	Six pieces	2 protein 1 carbohydrate 1 fat
Chicken wings, spicy	Six pieces (5 ounces)	6 protein 1 carbohydrate 1½ fat
Chicken salad	1 cup (8 ounces)	2 protein ½ carbohydrate 1 fat
Cream-style soup, made with water	1 cup (8 ounces)	1 carbohydrate 1 fat
Fish sandwich, with tartar sauce	One sandwich	1 protein 3 carbohydrate 3 fat
French fries	A medium-size carton (5 ounces)	4 carbohydrate 4 fat
Frozen dinner, with fewer than 340 calories	7 to 11 ounces	1 to 2 protein 2 to 3 carbohydrate
Hamburger with bun, regular size	One burger	2 protein 2 carbohydrate

Hamburger with bun, large	One burger	2 protein 2 carbohydrate 1 fat
Hot dog with bun	One hot dog	1 protein 1 carbohydrate 1 fat
Lasagna with meat	1 cup (8 ounces)	2 protein 2 carbohydrate
Macaroni and cheese	1 cup (8 ounces)	2 protein 2 carbohydrate
Pizza, thin crust cheese	One fourth of a 12-inch pie (6 ounces)	2 protein 2 carbohydrate 1½ fat
Pizza, thin crust meat	One half of a 12-inch pie (6 ounces)	2 protein 2 carbohydrate 1½ fat
Pizza, personal	One 6-inch pie	3 protein 5 carbohydrate 3 fat
Pot pie *Chicken or turkey*	One 6-inch pie (7 ounces)	1 protein 2½ carbohydrate 3 fat
Spaghetti with meatballs	1 cup (8 ounces)	2 protein 2 carbohydrate
Split pea soup made with water	½ cup (4 ounces)	1 carbohydrate
Submarine sandwich, regular size	One sandwich (6 inches)	2 protein 3½ carbohydrate 1 fat
Submarine sandwich, low-fat	One sandwich (6 inches)	2 protein 3 carbohydrate
Taco, hard or soft shell	One taco	1 protein 1 carbohydrate 1 fat
Tomato soup, made with water	1 cup (8 ounces)	1 carbohydrate
Tuna casserole	1 cup (8 ounces)	2 protein 2 carbohydrate
Tuna salad	1 cup (8 ounces)	2 protein ½ carbohydrate 1 fat

Fats

Fat servings should only be eaten in the morning, with breakfast. Fat helps provide satiety (though not nearly as well as protein) but needs to be included only at breakfast so your body can process it appropriately. Note: Foods marked with an asterisk (*) are unsaturated fats; foods without are saturated fats.

SHORTENING AND SPREADS

	ONE SERVING EQUALS
Butter	1 teaspoon
Butter, reduced-fat	1 tablespoon
Butter, whipped	2 teaspoons
Cream cheese	1 tablespoon
Cream cheese, reduced-fat	4½ teaspoons
Sour cream	2 tablespoons
Sour cream, reduced-fat	3 tablespoons
Cream, heavy (whipping)	1 tablespoon
Cream, half-and-half	2 tablespoons
Nondairy cream	2 tablespoons
Nondairy powdered coffee creamer	4 teaspoons
Shortening or lard	1 teaspoon
*__Margarine,__ reduced-fat	1 tablespoon
*__Mayonnaise__	1 teaspoon
*__Mayonnaise,__ reduced-fat	1 tablespoon
*__Miracle Whip dressing__	2 teaspoons
*__Miracle Whip dressing,__ reduced-fat	1 tablespoon
*__Tartar Sauce__	1 tablespoon
*__Tartar Sauce,__ reduced-fat	2 tablespoons

OILS AND
SALAD DRESSINGS

ONE SERVING EQUALS

*Oil
Including olive, vegetable, corn, canola,
peanut, sesame, and coconut oil   1 teaspoon

Salad dressing, creamy reduced-fat   1 teaspoon

Salad dressing, creamy fat-free   1 tablespoon

Salad dressing, Italian fat-free   1 tablespoon

Salad dressing, vinaigrette   2 tablespoons

NUTS AND SEEDS

ONE SERVING EQUALS

*Almonds, dry roasted or raw   Four to six almonds

*Almond butter, smooth or crunchy   1½ teaspoons
(also counts as
½ serving of meat)

*Peanuts, shelled   Ten large peanuts

*Peanut butter, smooth or crunchy   1½ teaspoons
(also counts as
½ serving of meat)

*Walnuts   Four walnut halves

*Other nuts
Including cashews and pecans   Four to six whole nuts

*Sunflower seeds, shelled   2 tablespoons

*Pumpkin seeds   4 tablespoons

*Sesame Seeds   1 tablespoon

*Tahini   2 teaspoons

OTHER FATS

ONE SERVING EQUALS

*Avocado   One eighth of a small
avocado (2 tablespoons)

Coconut, shredded   2 tablespoons

Coconut, milk	¼ cup
*Olives, ripe black	8 large olives
*Olives, green	10 large olives

Condiments

Used in moderation, condiments can add interest to meals—spoon up a dash of salsa to spice up tacos, spread a dollop of mustard on your sandwich for a touch of flavor, or pour a bit of syrup over your pancakes at breakfast. Reserve the sweeter condiments for breakfast and avoid them altogether at dinner.

	ONE SERVING EQUALS
Barbecue sauce	2 tablespoons
Cocktail sauce	2 tablespoons
Jam or jelly, low-sugar or sugar-free	2 tablespoons
Ketchup	1 tablespoon
Mustard	1 tablespoon
Pancake syrup, sugar-free	2 tablespoons
Pickles, sweet bread-and-butter	Two slices
Pickles, dill	One and one-half large pickles
Pickles, gherkin	¾ ounce
Pickle relish	1 tablespoon
Salsa	¼ cup
Soy sauce, regular or reduced-sodium	1 tablespoon
Sweet-and-sour sauce	1 tablespoon
Teriyaki sauce	1 tablespoon

Free Foods

There are beverages that you can consume throughout the day that don't count toward your meal servings. There are also a wide variety of seasonings you can use to spark up the flavors in the dishes you prepare.

BEVERAGES

Club soda

Coffee, regular or decaffeinated
Unsweetened or with sugar substitute (drink only after breakfast)

Diet soda, sugar-free

Powdered drink mixes, sugar-free

Tea,
Unsweetened or with sugar substitute (drink only after breakfast)

Tonic water, sugar-free

Water, plain, carbonated, or mineral

Water, flavored sugar-free

SEASONINGS

Butter flavoring, fat-free

Flavored extracts
Including almond, peppermint, and vanilla

Garlic

Herbs

Horseradish

Hot pepper sauce

Lemon juice
Use only after breakfast.

Lime juice
Use only after breakfast.

Pepper, ground

Pimentos

Salt

Spices

Vinegar

Wine
Use only for cooking.

Worcestershire sauce

OTHER

Bouillon, broth, and consommé, fat-free

Chewing gum, sugar-free

Cooking oil spray

Gelatin, unflavored or sugar-free

Sugar substitutes,
Including Splenda

FRUIT AND VEGETABLE LISTS

On my Big Breakfast Diet plan, you'll eat a fair amount of fruits and vegetables at lunch and dinner. But since your body's ability to use insulin starts to wane by midday, you need to be mindful of the sugar content in each serving of these fruits and vegetables. Some contain very little, less than 5 percent per serving, while others pack 15 to 20 percent per serving or even more. The general rule is: The less sugar per serving that fruits and vegetables contain, the more of them you can eat. For example, watermelon is very sweet, but actually contains less sugar per serving than strawberries or kiwifruit.

You can enjoy any and all fruits and vegetables, as long as you eat the recommended amounts. Feel free to mix and match from the vegetable and fruit groups—try any combination that appeals to you. Not only will you get to enjoy your favorites, you're bound to discover new combinations that please your eyes and your palate. For example, try combining three stalks of grilled asparagus with a quarter cup each of cauliflower and eggplant. Delicious!

Vegetables

1 serving = 2 grams protein, 5 grams carbohydrate, 0 grams fat, and 25 calories

VEGETABLE GROUP A

Less than 5% sugar per serving; 1 serving = 1 cup, raw, steamed, grilled, or roasted or as noted

Artichokes

Asparagus,
7 stalks

Bell peppers,
any color

Bok Choy

Broccoli

Cabbage or sauerkraut

Cauliflower

Celery

Collards

Cucumber

Eggplant

Greens
*Lettuce, sprouts, watercress,
and other salad greens*

Kale

Mushrooms

Radishes

Scallions or chives

Spinach, regular or baby

Tomatoes

Tomato sauce,
½ cup

Water chestnuts

Zucchini and
yellow summer squash

VEGETABLE GROUP B

5 to 10% sugar per serving; 1 serving = ½ cup, raw, steamed, grilled, or roasted or as noted

Beans, string or green

Beets

Brussels sprouts

Carrots

Corn, on the cob,
1 small ear

Corn, on the cob,
½ small ear

Green peas

Onions, white or red

Pumpkin or winter squash
*Including acorn, butternut,
and Hubbard squash*

Snow peas

Turnips and parsnips

Yams or sweet potatoes

Fruit

1 serving = 0 grams protein, 15 grams carbohydrate, 0 grams fat, and 60 calories

FRUIT GROUP A

Less than 5% sugar per serving as noted

Cantaloupe
⅓ small melon (1 cup cubed)

Cranberries, dried,
sweetened with sugar substitute

Guava
1 medium-size

Honeydew
⅛ medium-size melon (1 cup cubed)

Passion fruit
3 medium-size

Watermelon
1 generous cup cubed

FRUIT GROUP B
5 to 10% sugar per serving; 1 serving as noted

Grapefruit, ½ large

Grapefruit juice, ½ cup

Kiwifruit, 1 whole

Kumquats, 5 medium-size

Orange, 1 small

Orange juice, ½ cup

Papaya, ½ medium-size (1 cup)

Strawberries, 1¼ cups

Tangelo, 1 medium-size

Tangerines, 2 small

Tangerine juice, ½ cup

FRUIT GROUP C
10 to 15% sugar per serving; 1 serving as noted

Apple, 1 small

Apple juice, ½ cup

Apricots, 2 medium-size

Blackberries, ¾ cup

Blueberries, ¾ cup

Grapes, 17 small (3 ounces)

Grape juice, ⅓ cup

Mango, ½ small

Nectarine, 1 small

Peach, 1 medium-size

Pear, ½ large

Pineapple, fresh, ¾ cup cubed

Pineapple juice, ½ cup

Plums, 2 small

Pomegranate, ½ medium-size

Raspberries, 1 cup

FRUIT GROUP D
15 to 20% sugar or more per serving; 1 serving as noted

Apples, dried, 4 rings

Apricots, dried, 8 halves

Banana, ½ large

Cherries, fresh, 12

Cherries, canned, ½ cup

Dates, 3 medium-size

Figs, fresh, 2 medium-size

Figs, dried, 1½ medium-size

Prunes, 3 medium-size

Prune juice, ⅓ cup

Raisins, 2 tablespoons

Breakfast Sweets

Satisfy your sweet tooth in the morning with any of these foods and eliminate cravings later in the day.

ONE SERVING EQUALS

Animal crackers	Eight animal crackers
Brownie	One 2-inch square
Cake, frosted or unfrosted	One 2 inch–square slice
Cake, angel food	One 1½ inch–thick slice
Chocolate mint patty	One patty
Chocolate bar, plain, with almonds, or with rice crisps	1½ ounces
Chocolate kisses, plain or with almonds	Six kisses
Cookies	Two small cookies
Doughnut	One small cake doughnut
Frozen yogurt	⅓ cup
Frozen yogurt, fat-free	½ cup
Gingersnaps	Three gingersnaps
Graham crackers	Three 2 inch–square crackers
Ice cream, fat-free, no sugar added	½ cup
Jelly beans	14 jelly beans
Jelly beans, sugar-free	25 jelly beans
M&M's, plain	1½ ounces
M&M's, peanut	1¾ ounces
Muffin	One small muffin
Peanut butter cups	Four miniature peanut butter cups

Pudding, sweetened with sugar	¼ cup
Pudding, sugar-free	½ cup
Quick bread *Including banana, pumpkin, and zucchini bread*	One ⅜ inch–thick slice
Sherbet and sorbet	¼ cup
Snickers bar	One ¾-ounce-bar
Strawberry twists	2½ ounces
Vanilla wafers	Five vanilla wafers

THE BIG BREAKFAST DIET CURE

L et's try a little test. What did you have for breakfast this morning?

1. Doughnut-shop fare: muffin, bagel, or doughnut with coffee
2. Fast-food breakfast: heavy on the biscuits and hash browns
3. Diner fare: Eggs, waffles or pancakes, bacon or sausage, hash browns
4. Health-conscious options: cereal or oatmeal, yogurt, fruit
5. None of the above (Who can eat before noon?)

Regardless of your answer, you can take one simple step to make a dramatic difference in your weight: Give your morning meal a makeover. If you typically don't eat breakfast, it's time to start. (Don't panic, don't stop reading—just take a deep breath and check out page 82 for painless ways to get into the breakfast habit.)

THE SKINNY

Research shows that breakfast eaters tend to weigh less than breakfast skippers. Research also shows that some foods promote satiety better than others, and those are the ones to include in your morning meal. Learn to follow the Breakfast Formula on page 75 to create your own tasty morning meals, or use any of the 10 sample breakfasts in chapter 6 (pages 106 through 116).

It's worth it. Studies conducted on eating habits suggest that eating breakfast regularly can:

▶ Reduce risk of high cholesterol and insulin resistance,
▶ Minimize impulsive snacking and overeating at other meals, and
▶ Reduce the risk of overweight and obesity.

Research has long shown that people who eat breakfast tend to be slimmer than those who skip it. Adults who skip breakfast are likely to take in more calories during the course of the day than people who do eat breakfast.

One compelling study was conducted by the National Weight Control Registry (NWCR). Formed by obesity researchers at Brown Medical School and the University of Colorado, the NWCR is the largest study of people who have managed to keep off the weight they've lost. In this 2002 study, conducted by the University of Colorado Health Sciences Center in Denver, researchers surveyed a group of 2,959 men and women who'd lost 30 pounds or more and kept it off for at least a year. Some had maintained their weight loss for as long as six years. They found that 78 percent reported eating breakfast every day. Almost 90 percent said they ate it at least five days a week. Interestingly, the breakfast eaters and breakfast skippers consumed almost the same total daily calories; the breakfast skippers made up the missed breakfast calories throughout the day. In addition, researchers at the University of Massachusetts Medical School found that breakfast skippers are 4.5 times more likely to be obese than are breakfast eaters.

Recall that eating breakfast sends a message to your brain and body that all is well; that it won't starve today; that it's okay to burn glucose for energy, because more is on the way.

That said, if you want to lose weight, some breakfast options are better than others. My research showed that women who followed my breakfast plan revved their metabolism; reduced their cravings for sweets and starches, which typically hit from midafternoon on; and felt satiated all day.

In this chapter, you'll learn the breakfast plan that turbocharges weight loss—without hunger or cravings. The fact is, some foods promote that satisfying, "I'm full" feeling more than others do (see The Satiety Index, page 86), and those are the foods to include in your morning meal.

Hunger, Hormones, and Satiety

Ever said "I'm hungry" just a few hours after you've eaten a meal? Most likely, what you're describing is appetite, the psychological *desire* to eat. Appetite is triggered by your senses—which are stimulated by seeing, smelling, or tasting food—or by your emotions, as when you recall a past pleasant experience with food.

By contrast, hunger is a physiological *need* for food. When you're hungry, you experience physical symptoms: Your stomach rumbles, or you feel tired, moody, or mentally fuzzy. These signals are your body's way of demanding that you provide it with nourishment.

Both hunger and satiety are regulated by the hypothalamus gland. Hormonal messages that pass between the hypothalamus and the digestive system either increase hunger, signaling to the brain that the body needs food, or increase satiety, telling the brain that eating should stop because the stomach is full.

When your body needs food, the hypothalamus detects changing levels of hormones released in your stomach, gut, and body fat and transmits a message: "Eat!" If you ignore this message, the brain becomes alarmed and produces a variety of chemicals designed to wipe out all other thoughts and desires but those for food.

Perhaps the hunger hormone that has been studied the most is ghrelin. Secreted by special cells in the stomach wall, ghrelin activates hunger-related neurotransmitters in the brain, effectively telling the brain it's time to eat. Levels of ghrelin in our blood rise gradually before a meal, which signals the hypothalamus to release chemicals that trigger eating (such as neuropeptide Y). Immediately after we eat, ghrelin levels fall. Ghrelin levels don't fall as much in the evening as they do during the day. This explains why people who have their largest meal at dinner, rather than at breakfast, may feel hungry later in the night.

When you eat and become full, your hormone levels change again, and the hypothalamus sends a different message: "Stop eating." (It takes about 20 minutes for your brain to get the "I'm full" signal to your stomach.) In several hours, when the stomach empties, you'll feel hungry again.

The best-known "satiety hormone" is leptin. Made by fat cells, leptin signals the brain that the body has enough energy stores, such as body fat. Other satiety hormones include the digestive hormone cholecystokinin (CCK) and glucagon-like peptide-1 (GLP-1). Both CCK and GLP-1 are known to enhance satiety and cause the stomach to empty its contents more slowly, which results in that "I'm full" feeling.

How the Big Breakfast Turns On Weight Loss, Turns Off Hunger and Cravings

It's very possible to eat a large breakfast that leaves you hungry the whole day. If you eat foods that have a weak ability to diminish hunger, the big breakfast won't do you any good. But my breakfast contains two types of foods that research has shown promote satiety:

▶ Protein foods
▶ Carbohydrate foods with a low glycemic index (GI)

THE BIG BREAKFAST DIET
BREAKFAST FORMULA

▶ 7 servings protein (2 of which must be milk- or yogurt-based, see page 54)
▶ 2 servings carbohydrate
▶ 2 servings fat
▶ 1 serving Breakfast Sweet

PROTEINS: 7 SERVINGS
Wards Off Hunger, Revs Up Metabolism

Studies show that overweight people experience more frequent food cravings, and less satiety, even when they eat adequate amounts of food. But take heart; research suggests that eating more high-quality protein—low-fat milk or yogurt, fish, lean red meat or poultry—while consuming fewer carbohydrates and saturated fats can help reduce the total number of calories eaten each day. This is because, according to research findings, protein—rather than carbohydrate or fat—most promotes satiety.

What's more, people who eat a diet moderate in carbohydrates and high in protein increase their chances of maintaining weight loss over time.

Research suggests that protein fills you up sooner and wards off hunger longer than carbs—and those who eat a higher-protein diet tend to agree. In a 2005 study published in the *American Journal of Clinical Nutrition,* people who followed a 30 percent protein diet ate 441 fewer calories per day than when they followed a diet that contained only 15 percent protein.

Another provocative finding about satiety is that clinical studies have shown that the more people eat in the morning, the less they tend to eat throughout the day. The more they eat at night, the more calories they take in overall.

In one small but interesting 2006 study of 15 men, a high-protein breakfast reduced blood levels of ghrelin more effectively than did a high-carbohydrate breakfast.

In another study, conducted in 2008, researchers at Purdue University put two groups of overweight men on a reduced-calorie diet. One group consumed a normal amount of protein (11 to 14 percent of daily calories) and the other group, a larger amount (18 to 25 percent of daily calories). The researchers tested the effect of consuming the additional protein at specific meals (breakfast, lunch, *or* dinner)—or spaced evenly throughout the day (breakfast, lunch, *and* dinner). The study found that only protein eaten at breakfast contributed to a greater sense of satiety throughout the day.

There's still an element of mystery as to why a higher-protein diet satisfies hunger so well. In the Purdue study, the researchers found that the higher-protein diet enhanced the effect of leptin, the satiety hormone. Interestingly, however, this diet also caused ghrelin levels to rise, which should, in theory, *increase* appetite. Instead, the men were *less* hungry!

Bear in mind that consuming the servings of protein I recommend should keep your hunger at bay for up to 14 hours. If you're ravenous by noon, you probably filled up on too many starches at breakfast and skimped on protein.

THE ROLE OF MILK:
WHY IT'S SO IMPORTANT

To succeed on the Big Breakfast Diet plan, you must drink two cups of nonfat milk or soy milk in the morning. Why? Because both dairy milk and soy milk are good sources of high-quality protein, which controls hunger. Milk also contains nutrients that accelerate metabolism. In fact, women who drink more milk tend to burn more calories, according to research conducted at Purdue University: Calcium reduces parathyroid hormone, which in turn increases fat burning.

While two cups seems like a lot, consider this: You're in control of when and how you consume it. You can drink one cup with 3 tablespoons of whey in a shake or smoothie. Or, if you prefer, you can have one cup in a shake or smoothie (without whey) with one cup in your cereal later at work, as long as you finish your breakfast by 9 A.M. (or 10 A.M. in fall and winter).

If you're lactose-intolerant and milk leaves you gassy, crampy, and bloated, try drinking milk made for people with lactose intolerance or opt for soy milk.

CARBOHYDRATES: 2 SERVINGS
Low Is the Way to Go

All carbohydrates are not created equal. While some carbohydrate foods cause blood sugar and insulin levels to spike, others have little impact on blood sugar and insulin. The glycemic index (GI) ranks foods by how they affect your blood sugar (see pages 87–89). Specifically, the GI measures how much a 50-gram portion of a carbohydrate (a bit less than 2 ounces) raises blood sugar compared to pure glucose, which has a "score" of 100.

Your body digests low-GI foods (ranked less than 55) slowly, which produces a slow, gentle rise in blood sugar and insulin. The lower on this scale the foods you eat, the better it is for your health and weight. A recent study in *The Journal of the American Medical Association* found that people with type 2 diabetes who ate a low-GI diet for six months had greater blood sugar control and fewer heart disease risk factors than those who didn't. Research has found that people who eat a lot of low-GI foods tend to have lower levels of body fat.

Most fruits, vegetables, legumes, and whole grains—of which you'll be eating a lot on this plan—are low-GI foods, in large part because their high fiber content slows digestion. (I'm sure you'll be pleased to note that dark chocolate is a low-GI food.)

Foods that rank between 55 and 70 are moderate-GI foods; the foods your body digests and absorbs rapidly are high-GI foods and rank over 70. High-GI foods include bread, rice, pasta, and baked goods.

Swapping high-GI foods for those that rank low to moderate on the index keeps blood sugar and insulin levels more stable. This in turn controls hunger and makes it easier for your body to lose fat. When you're building your meals, it helps to be mindful of the

GI of your ingredients. For example, if you are preparing a bean dish for breakfast and have a choice of canned beans, choose red kidney beans or white beans because they have a lower GI than baked beans.

Whole (unprocessed), high-fiber foods tend to have lower GI scores, but there are exceptions. Some foods, including carrots, potatoes, rice, and pasta, can either be high- or low-GI foods, depending on how long they're cooked, among other factors. The ripeness of a fruit or veggie also plays a role: The riper it is, the higher its GI score. Some junk foods have surprisingly low GI scores, whereas some healthy foods, such as rice cakes, have a high GI.

You can use the glycemic index to guide your food selections. While the goal is to choose mostly low- and moderate-GI foods, use your common sense. Select whole foods such as fruits, veggies, legumes, and whole grains as often as possible—and make sure you eat those chips and doughnuts for breakfast.

FATS: 2 SERVINGS
Quality over Quantity

Dietary fat isn't all bad. Your body uses the fats in food for energy. Dietary fat also helps promote satiety (although not as much as protein) and helps your body absorb fat-soluble vitamins, including vitamins D and E. Your body also uses the fats in food to make hormonelike substances that help regulate blood pressure and heart rate, among other vital functions.

Some dietary fats are better for your body than others. Plant foods (fruits and vegetables) and fish are sources of *healthy, unsaturated* fats. *Unhealthy, saturated* fats are found in animal foods, including beef, pork, lard, butter, and dairy products made from whole and 2 percent milk. (These foods, along with egg yolks, also contain dietary cholesterol.) Saturated fats are the main diet-related cause of high blood cholesterol, and diets high in saturated fats are linked with several chronic diseases, including heart disease. (See box below for the American Heart Association's guidelines for dietary fat.)

Trans fats, typically found in commercially baked foods and baked fried goods (crackers, cookies, cakes, doughnuts, French fries), can raise blood cholesterol even more than saturated fats. Fortunately, food companies have taken steps to reduce the trans fats in their products.

Eating large amounts of fat, whether unsaturated or saturated, means you consume more calories, which can lead to overweight and obesity. (Fat contains 9 calories per gram, compared with 4 calories per gram for protein and carbohydrates.)

Choose your breakfast fats from the table in chapter 3. Most of your dietary fat should come from healthy monounsaturated and polyunsaturated fats, which include vegetable oils, nuts and nut butters, olives, and avocados. If you have elevated blood cholesterol, limit egg yolks to two per week (egg whites contain no cholesterol) and opt for low-fat and fat-free dairy products.

EAT LESS FAT, WEAR LESS FAT

Follow the American Heart Association's dietary fat guidelines in conjunction with the Big Breakfast Diet program and you'll reap a double benefit: better health and less body fat.

Total fat: less than 25–35 percent of total calories each day
Saturated fat: less than 7 percent of total daily calories
Trans fat: less than 1 percent of total daily calories
Dietary cholesterol: less than 300 mg per day, for most people

THE BREAKFAST SWEET: 1 SERVING
Have Your Chocolate—Doctor's Orders

Many of my patients have told me that the "breakfast sweet" is one of the most enjoyable parts of their day, and not just because they look forward to their doughnut, piece of cake, or dish of pudding. It's because, for perhaps the first time ever, their guilt about eating sweets is gone. Never before have they been told that it's okay, even necessary, to indulge their sweet tooth on a diet. That they must enjoy their treat in the morning takes some getting used to, but they soon adjust.

A few of my patients told me that they just didn't believe that eating a doughnut, or a piece of cake, in the morning would reduce their desire for sweets later on. Their skepticism vanished after a day or so—as did their uncontrollable afternoon or evening yen for chocolate.

We're talking simple brain chemistry: If you eat sweets in the morning, serotonin levels stay elevated throughout the day. By preventing an aggressive serotonin nosedive in the afternoon (which would cause sluggishness and irritability) you're successfully fending off cravings, too.

What's interesting is that when you eat a sweet in the morning, you won't be "rewarded" with that sense of calm, even euphoria, you may experience when you eat it in the afternoon or evening. You simply eat the chocolate or the cheese Danish, enjoy it, and forget about sweets until the next morning. When you keep your serotonin levels where they should be—and remove the association between sweets and positive mood—you begin to break the addiction.

Choose any sweet from the table in chapter 3. Never, ever skip your sweet to "save calories." Just as proteins control hunger, sweets control carbohydrate addiction.

Help for Those Who Hate Breakfast

It takes most of my breakfast skippers about a week to get used to their morning meal. But after that, few of them ever pass up breakfast again—they feel too good. Not only have they lost weight or maintained their loss, but they have more energy at work; their minds are sharper, their moods brighter. They get into a positive spiral—the more days they eat a big breakfast, the better they feel.

BREAKFAST NOTES

▶ If you're running short on time, select one of the four Dine and Dash meals, marked with an arrow ( ), starting on page 107.

▶ You must eat *at least* seven servings of protein. (You don't want to be starving by lunch, do you?) You can eat more protein if you wish, but never less.

▶ Unless indicated, all smoothies or shakes are prepared with 8 ounces of skim milk or plain low-fat yogurt along with 3 tablespoons of whey, so you can get your two servings of milk quickly and easily.

▶ You may use an artificial sweetener, such as Splenda.

▶ The sample breakfasts are just examples. Use the Big Breakfast Diet Servings List, starting on page 54, to "build" any meal you like, as long as it follows the formula. That means you can have a bacon cheeseburger for breakfast: four or five meat servings with one to two cheese servings will net you your seven servings of protein. Add two slices of bacon for your fat servings. The bun delivers your carb servings. Plus, you still get to enjoy your smoothie or shake and breakfast sweet!

▶ If you can't eat your entire breakfast at one sitting, don't worry, you don't have to. Simply split it into two or three servings and finish them all by 9 A.M. (or 10 A.M. in the fall and winter).

On the rare days when they're too rushed to eat, or eat less protein than they should, they feel foggy and out of sorts. The very next day, they're back on the breakfast bandwagon.

If you dislike eating in the morning, let me ask you: How badly do you want to lose weight? If you're willing to give my method a try, I can promise that you will get used to your morning meal and even look forward to it.

Here's the simplest way to "learn" to eat breakfast: Break your meal into two or even three parts until you adjust to eating in the morning.

First, sip an 8-ounce Shake or Smoothie (see pages 50 to 52). This mini-meal gives your brain the glucose it needs to function and prevents it from activating its morning emergency system. Then eat the rest of your breakfast, say, half a bagel with smoked salmon and cream cheese and an 8-ounce glass of milk, by 9 A.M. Be patient—in a week or so, you'll likely look forward to your morning meal.

The Satiety Index

More than a decade ago, Susanne Holt, Ph.D., and her colleagues at the University of Sydney in Australia had volunteers eat a 240-calorie portion of 33 different foods. Then they asked the volunteers to rate their feelings of hunger every 15 minutes over a two-hour period. During these two hours, the researchers gave the volunteers access to a buffet table of food. They were allowed to eat their fill, as the team watched.

The researchers gave white bread a baseline score of 100. Foods with a score higher than 100 were judged to be more satisfying than white bread; those that scored less than 100 were less satisfying. Voila! The Satiety Index (SI) was born. Continue reading to learn what the researchers found.

A NEW KIND OF
BREAKFAST SANDWICH

If you love your eggs and bacon, by all means, enjoy! But if you want to eat like one of my patients in South America, you'll opt for ... a sandwich.

Before you wrinkle your nose at the prospect, let me explain. First, eggs are the least satiating of the proteins. Second, a sandwich will fill you up. Third, sandwiches are incredibly easy to make. My patients are constantly telling me they don't have time for breakfast, but how long does it take to make a sandwich? Five to ten minutes, tops. Even better, once you make it, you can eat it on the run. (And it's a lot easier to eat a sandwich in the car than a bowl of cereal or a plate of scrambled eggs!)

Most important, sandwiches are the simplest way to get the protein-fat-carb combo that's the cornerstone of the Big Breakfast Diet plan.

Bread is the foundation of any good sandwich. If you want to stick with your everyday sliced sandwich bread, no problem. But you have many other choices, including the following:

▶ High-SI foods—baked potatoes, popcorn, high-fiber cereals—are bulky and high in fiber, which means that they require a lot of chewing and swallowing. These actions help the body recognize that it's full.

▶ High-SI foods such as oatmeal and apples help block absorption of fat and calories because they're high in fiber, which contains no calories, and because fiber speeds food out of the body.

▶ Compared to low-SI foods, high-SI foods provide more energy from lean protein sources, including fish, beef, eggs, cheese, and beans.

- ▶ Half a small to medium bagel
- ▶ Corn bread
- ▶ Italian bread
- ▶ Focaccia
- ▶ Hard roll

- ▶ Flour or corn tortillas
- ▶ Pita bread
- ▶ French baguette
- ▶ Cinnamon-raisin bread

Now for the filling options:

- ▶ Lean cold cuts: smoked ham or turkey, roast beef
- ▶ Pastrami or corned beef
- ▶ Cheese

- ▶ Fish: smoked lox on half a crusty bagel with cream cheese!
- ▶ Nut butters: peanut, almond, or sunflower

An important part of any sandwich are the "extras": things like veggies, condiments (the traditional mustard or ketchup, or salsa, hummus, or tahini spread), and even fresh or dried fruit. Since this is breakfast, feel free to use ketchup, mustard, margarine, cream cheese, and mayo (in the recommended amounts, see pages 62 and 64) along with any of the fixings you'd enjoy in a sandwich shop—lettuce, tomatoes, onions, cucumbers, hot or sweet peppers, salsa, and fresh or dried herbs and spices.

Remember to stick to the portion sizes on pages 54–70.

The researchers' conclusion? A diet based on high-SI foods can help people trying to lose weight reduce the number of calories they consume *without* having to severely curtail their food intake or deal with extreme hunger between meals.

The Satiety Index that follows is a guide to just some of the foods you are likely to include in your diet. Note: These foods are ranked *only* by the satisfaction that a 240-calorie serving offers (so the kind of doughnut or cookie you have is only limited by its serving size). However, the Satiety Index does help you understand how much more filling certain foods are (cookies) than others (a slice of cake).

SATIETY INDEX

The sampling of foods below is based on 240-calorie servings.
Foods with higher scores satisfy your hunger better.

PROTEIN-RICH FOODS

Lentils	133
Cheese	146
Eggs	150
Baked beans	168
Beef	176
Ling fish	225

CARBOHYDRATE-RICH FOODS

White bread	100
French fries	116
White pasta	119
Brown rice	132
White rice	138
Whole-grain bread	154
Whole-meal bread	157
Whole-grain pasta	188
Potatoes, boiled	323

CEREALS WITH MILK (WHOLE)

Müesli	100
Special K	116
Cornflakes	118
Honey Smacks	132
All-Bran	151
Oatmeal	209

FRUIT

Bananas	118
Grapes	162
Apples	197
Oranges	202

BAKED GOODS

Plain croissant	47
Cake slice	65
Doughnuts (240-calorie serving)	68
Cookies (240-calorie serving)	120
Crackers	127

CANDY AND SNACKS

Mars bar	70
Peanuts	84
Yogurt	88
Potato chips	91
Ice cream	96
Jellybeans	118
Popcorn	154

---

*Adapted from S.H.A. Holt, J. C. Brand Miller, P. Petocz, and E. Farmakalidis,
"A Satiety Index of Common Foods,"* European Journal of Clinical Nutrition,
September 1995, pages 675–690.

GLYCEMIC INDEX

A food's glycemic index (GI) score measures the rate at which that food is broken down by the body and converted into glucose—in other words, how fast you get that sugar rush after you've eaten. High-GI foods score greater than 70, low-GI foods score less than 55, and moderate-GI foods rank in between. Foods with high-GI make your glucose level spike and then swiftly drop, causing you to feel hungry again soon after eating; foods with low-GI are digested more slowly, keeping your glucose level steady and maintaining a feeling of fullness longer.

You can reduce the rush from high-sugar foods by eating them in the morning, in combination with other foods (which is why eating a Breakfast Sweet is mandatory!). Blood sugar and glycogen levels tend to be lower at that time, so your body will more likely store carbs as muscle and liver glycogen, rather than body fat. Interestingly, though both a baked potato and French fries have relatively high scores, fries rate lower than a baked potato, because the oil that they are cooked in slows down the absorption of glucose.

The list below includes just a sampling of common carbohydrate and starch sources that are appropriate to eat *only in the morning*, with your big breakfast.

BREADS

White bread	70	Dinner roll	73
Whole-wheat or whole-grain bread	69	Biscuit	75
		Croissant	67
Pumpernickel	41	Bagel	72
Rye bread	76	Hamburger or hot dog bun	62
French or Italian bread	95	Pita	57
		Taco shells	68

Corn tortillas	69
Corn bread or corn muffin	69
Muffin, plain	46
Muffin, bran	60
Muffin, banana, oat, or honey	65
Muffin, apple	44
Muffin, blueberry	59

CRACKERS AND SNACK FOODS

Soda crackers	74
Whole-wheat crackers	67
Rye crispbread	64
Rice crackers	91
Rice cakes	82
Melba toast	70
Pretzels	83
Chips, potato	55
Chips, tortilla	72
Chips, pita	57
Popcorn	55
Protein bar, peanut butter	22
Protein bar, chocolate-chip	30
Protein bar, chocolate	38
Protein bar, white chocolate	40
Protein bar, strawberry	43

CEREAL AND GRAINS

Puffed wheat	67
Puffed rice	81
Shredded wheat	67
Corn flakes	84
Bran cereal	54
Raisin bran	61
Oat bran	50
Honey nut cereal	74
Sugar-frosted cereal	51
Granola	43
Grape-Nuts	66
Müesli	49
Oatmeal	49
Grits	68
Rice, white long-grain	56
Rice, white short-grain	72
Buckwheat	54
Brown rice	55
Noodles	46
Bulgur	48
Couscous	65
Barley	43

PASTA AND OTHER STARCHES

| Spaghetti | 43 |
| Spaghetti, whole grain | 41 |

Spiral pasta	43
Macaroni	47
Fettuccini, egg	32
Ravioli, meat	39
Potato, boiled	70
Potato, baked	93
French fries	74

SWEETS

Pound cake	54
Banana cake	47
Chocolate cake with chocolate frosting	38
Strawberry cupcakes with frosting	73

Pastry	59
Doughnut	76
Vanilla wafers	78
Oatmeal cookies	55
Shortbread cookies	64
Chocolate mousse	63
Chocolate bar, milk	49
Chocolate bar, dark	23
Snickers bar	41
M&M's, plain	33
M&M's, peanut	32
Jelly beans	80

5

LUNCH

AND DINNER

A s you've learned, the hormones that transform food, especially foods rich in protein, into energy prevail in the morning, and by lunchtime, the body's hormonal landscape is in transition.

Insulin's ability to ferry glucose to the muscles for energy has fallen. Protein, which turbocharges metabolism when you eat it in the morning, has less effect on metabolism when consumed later in the day. The fat-burning hormone HGH will begin to rise by dinnertime.

To put it another way: In the morning cortisol and insulin run the show, and by evening the stage will be turned over to HGH. So at lunch, it's time to eat lean—a flank steak with a side of asparagus or broiled salmon with veggies.

You may not even want lunch, because the morning's tummy-satisfying protein will still be with you. Eat it anyway, to ensure that your hunger won't emerge full force later on. Dinner, on the other hand, is more flexible. If you're hungry, include up to three servings of protein. If not, enjoy lighter fare, without the protein servings.

One of the best things about the lunch and dinner formulas is their simplicity. It's easy to follow the plan, whether you eat in or dine out. If you tend to cook and eat at home, you'll spend minimal time in the kitchen. If you typically dine and dash, or if you enjoy eating out, you'll find plenty of lunch and dinner options at your local salad bar, chain restaurant, or the fanciest bistro in town. (Remember: You have the option of following the strict "turbocharged" version of my plan to lose weight quickly or the more relaxed option, which allows small amounts of oil and carbs later in the day but results in slower weight loss.)

A word about fruits and vegetables: You can have virtually any you desire. But because your body's ability to use insulin starts to wane by midday, be mindful of their sugar content. Some low-glycemic fruits and veggies contain very little sugar: less than 5 percent per serving. Others rank higher on the glycemic index and pack 15 to 20 percent per serving or even more. The less sugar per serving they contain, the more of them you can eat.

You won't feel limited as long as you pay attention to your Fruit and Vegetable Lists (pages 66 to 68) and consume the recommended amounts. For example, watermelon is very sweet,

THE SKINNY

Your afternoon and evening meals center around fruits and veggies, with a sensible portion of protein. You'll eat more fruit, which contains the greater amount of sugar, for lunch; and more veggies, which generally contain the smaller amount of sugar, at dinner.

For lunch and dinner, think *time* and *taste*. Both are vital to your enjoyment, and you'll learn plenty of easy ways to minimize preparation time and maximize flavor.

but it actually contains less sugar per serving than strawberries or kiwifruit, making it a smart choice for later in the day.

What's for Lunch?

If you typically eat a burger and fries, pizza, or other fast-food fare for lunch, prepare to be pleasantly surprised: If you've eaten your big breakfast, you simply won't want these "forbidden" foods. And if you do, you can eat them for breakfast tomorrow. Remember, on this plan, you focus not on calories but on eating the foods that satisfy your hunger and curb carbohydrate cravings at the time your body can best convert them to energy.

Here's your lunch formula:

PROTEINS: 3 SERVINGS

Select your nondairy proteins from the table starting on page 54. The less fat you use in the preparation of meat, poultry, and seafood, the faster the weight will come off. You may use a bit of cooking spray, or a couple teaspoons of olive oil, if you wish.

For a vegetarian lunch, you may enjoy unlimited veggie servings as well as another Smoothie or Shake (with 6 tablespoons of whey, not 3) to make sure you reach the appropriate satiety level at lunch. If you're vegan, opt for tofu or legumes, prepared with no or limited fat, or prepare The Smoothie with soy (including the increased whey servings).

VEGETABLES: 3 SERVINGS GROUP A, 2 SERVINGS GROUP B

Select your veggies from the table on page 66. Eat them any way you like—raw in salads, roasted, steamed, grilled, or sautéed. Again, the less fat (fewer oils) you use to prepare them, the more quickly you'll lose weight.

FEEL HUNGRY? CRAVE SWEETS?
CHECK YOUR BREAKFAST

The two central goals of this plan are to control hunger and manage carbohydrate addiction. If you experience either hunger or cravings at night, follow this advice.

IF YOU'RE HUNGRY AT NIGHT: Did you eat the recommended seven servings of proteins? If you did, eat more protein for breakfast—a few more slices of ham, turkey, or cheese, or a bit more tofu or tempeh. Continue to add protein until your night hunger stops.

IF YOU EXPERIENCE CARB CRAVINGS, BUT NOT HUNGER: Did you eat your breakfast sweet this morning, along with the recommended two servings of carbohydrates? If not, make sure to eat them tomorrow morning. If you did eat them, but still crave bread or cookies at night, hang in there. When you spend more time eating in sync, these "carb attacks" should fade.

FRUIT: 1 SERVING FROM GROUP A, B, C, OR D

Select your fruits from the table on page 67. The amount of fruit per serving depends on its sugar content. You can eat one, or you can mix several, as in a fruit cocktail or salad, calculating the amounts, especially for those that include more sugar.

Eat lunch before 2 P.M. (or 3 P.M. during Daylight Saving), and follow the formula below. For maximum weight loss, prepare your meal without fats or oils. However, at lunch, it is acceptable to use 1 to 2 tablespoons of healthy fats, such as olive oil, nuts, or seeds, or up to 2 tablespoons of low-calorie salad dressing.

If you typically buy lunch, it won't be hard to follow the formula. Hit the nearest salad bar and load up on lean proteins.

You can even eat at a fast-food place: Buy a burger, throw away the bun, and add a salad with low-calorie dressing.

It's Time for Dinner

For most of my patients, the most challenging aspect of my plan is not eating their largest meal at dinner and not snacking in the evening. It's challenging not because they're hungry, but because they're not used to watching TV, or going about their nightly routine, without eating.

Don't let these feelings throw you. It may take a day or two to adjust to eating in sync, but your mind will catch up with your body. And if you've followed the breakfast and lunch formulas, *you should not feel hungry.* All that protein you ate earlier in the day will make sure of that. Also, the sweets and starches you enjoyed at breakfast have kept your brain serotonin on an even keel, so you shouldn't experience cravings for them.

Follow this formula at dinner:

PROTEINS: 0 TO 3 SERVINGS

VEGETABLES: UNLIMITED SERVINGS GROUP A, 2 SERVINGS GROUP B

FRUIT: 1 SERVING GROUP A, 1 SERVING GROUP B

You'll notice that you can set your own servings of protein. If dinnertime rolls around and you're not hungry, congratulations! You've been following the formula right. Eat just the fruits and veggies (or, if you like, a bowl of veggie stew). If you do feel hungry, include the protein servings, but remember to add protein to your breakfast the following day—the goal is to eventually not be hungry in the evening.

If you're going out to dinner, try ordering a veggie plate. Some of my patients tell me that they add the protein "for show" when they dine out with business clients so they feel more a part of the festivities. You can follow this formula virtually anywhere—from the most inexpensive diner to the most elegant restaurant in town. No one in your party will notice if your dinner entrée is meat, veggies, and a salad—and you can always enjoy low-sugar fruit for dessert.

NEED A SNACK?
CURES FOR THE AFTERNOON
MUNCHIES

If you follow the Big Breakfast Diet plan (turbocharged or relaxed) to the letter and include the correct number of protein servings at breakfast and lunch, you should not feel hungry enough to require a snack in the afternoon or at night. However, if you absolutely need to snack, nosh on any of the "free foods" below, which can be consumed in unlimited amounts. See also the chart on page 65 for the full list.

- ▶ Raw or steamed vegetables, including cabbage, celery, cucumber, peppers, mushrooms, and radishes
- ▶ A bowl of The Stew, page 52
- ▶ Green salad made with lettuce, spinach, or endives
- ▶ Dried cranberries, artificially sweetened (½ cup, two to three times a day)
- ▶ Any artificially sweetened diet beverage (diet soft drinks, iced tea, powdered drink mix—preferably caffeine-free)
- ▶ Club soda, sugar-free tonic water, or carbonated water
- ▶ Coffee or tea (only in the afternoon)
- ▶ Sugar-free chewing gum

Eight Ways to Punch Up P.M. Meals

Remember when I said that my program was a way of life? I was sincere about that. The best way to stick to this way of eating for good is to expand your knowledge of food and cooking, to broaden your culinary horizons.

Pore through cookbooks. Explore vegetarian and vegan websites. Take field trips to specialty stores and farmers' markets. Compare organic produce to commercially grown fruits and vegetables. Your reward: a lean, healthy body and a new appreciation for food. Get inspired, get creative—and get started with these easy, practical tips.

WORK YOUR FRUIT. There's nothing healthier than a crisp, crunchy apple, but don't stop with whole fruit. Work with fruit the way an artist works with oils or watercolors. Try exotic fruits. In Venezuela, passionfruit and guava are quite common, but are less known in the United States. Combine low- and high-sugar fruits in fruit salads. Or if you love the taste of pink grapefruit,

CONSIDER PLATE APPEAL

When it comes to food, visual appeal is as important as taste. You might say we eat with our eyes. So as you prepare your lunches and dinners, consider that chefs study a technique called "plating" to make their creations as appealing to the eye as they are to the tastebuds.

Yes, sometimes you just want to get a healthy meal in your brown bag or on the dinner table. But you'll enjoy your meals more if you pay some attention to color, texture, and presentation. In fact, other cultures do this as a matter of routine.

tangerines, or other citrus fruits but not the pulp or white, stringy pith, squeeze them and enjoy their juice.

EXPAND YOUR DEFINITION OF "SALAD." Spinach salad is wonderful. So is the *insalata caprese* that Italians enjoy: thin slices of mozzarella, thick slices of tomato, and dried or fresh-cut basil and oregano. Or the Greek "village salad" of tomato, cucumber, and onion, drizzled with extra-virgin olive oil (if you're on the relaxed plan) and sprinkled with oregano, with or without tangy feta cheese.

SPOIL YOURSELF WITH BABY VEGGIES. Sweet to look at and sweeter to the taste, baby carrots, zucchini, and other miniature vegetables are as nutritious as their regular-size counterparts and most are more delicately flavored. You'll find them at larger grocery stores, specialty grocers, and farmers' markets.

SOUP UP YOUR VEGGIES. On a crisp fall or cold winter night, there's nothing tastier and more tummy-filling than pumpkin, tomato, or asparagus soup, prepared with a dash of low-fat milk and plenty

---

In Spain the practice of savoring small plates of a variety of small appetizers, called tapas, for a single meal is wildly popular. You can create your own tapas with a bit of fruit salad, a plate of grilled veggies, a chunk of good cheese, a dollop of tuna, or a slice of grilled meat or poultry. The variations are endless.

Or go Japanese with the bento, the traditional single-portion takeout or home-packed meal. Although traditional bento includes steamed rice, its other components are fish or meat and one or more vegetables, which is right in keeping with my program's recommendations. To ignite your imagination and your palate, search for cookbooks and websites devoted to both traditional bento and westernized, bento-inspired meals.

of herbs and spices. Search vegetarian websites for recipes. *Hint:*
Opt for vegetables that can be puréed, which ensures a thick,
hearty soup without the need for cream.

DISCOVER PLAIN, FAT-FREE GREEK YOGURT. Tangy, thick, and
creamy, it's an amazing substitute for mayonnaise or sour
cream—and a good source of calcium and protein to boot.
To whip up a creamy dip for veggies, blend with salt or salt
substitute, freshly ground pepper, spices, and fresh herbs. Mix
a dollop with a pinch of dried mustard or a bit of horseradish or
wasabi and use to top grilled fish or poultry, too.

EXPERIMENT WITH EXOTIC CONDIMENTS AND SPICES. Besides old
faithfuls like ketchup (only 1 tablespoon) and mustard, try chili
or wasabi, Indian curry paste, fresh horseradish or ginger root
(or prepared paste), capers, and cracked black pepper.

SPLURGE ON BALSAMIC VINEGAR. It's pricier than red, white, or
cider vinegars, because it's aged for a longer period. But the
longer it's aged, the thicker and more flavorful it gets. Drizzle
over cheese, steamed veggies, and greens, or add a tablespoon
or two to other dishes.

COOK WITH FIRE. Add curry, crushed red pepper, or cayenne to a
meal to give it exra flavor and kick. If you're not used to these
spices, use them sparingly—a tiny portion can pack a lot of heat.

Time: Make It Quick

Many of my patients have families and demanding jobs,
and don't have a lot of time to cook. Fortunately, most
supermarkets now offer a wide variety of prepared foods that
are also well suited to my lunch and dinner formulas. In fact,

FOR YOUR HEART
(AND WAISTLINE),
OPT FOR LEAN MEATS

While all meats contain saturated fat and dietary cholesterol, some contain less of these unhealthy fats than others do. Instead of using regular ground beef or fatty "prime cuts" of red meat, consider these leaner alternatives:

▶ poultry: turkey, Cornish game hen
▶ ground beef: lean or extra-lean (no more than 15 percent of calories from fat)
▶ pork: pork tenderloin, loin pork chop
▶ lamb: leg of lamb, arm of lamb, loin
▶ game: venison, buffalo, rabbit

buying prepared foods can help fend off temptation by keeping you out of the kitchen. With these quick-prep ideas, you can whip up tasty meals that even your family will love, in less time than you think.

Stock your kitchen with the staples. Along with the flavorful ingredients mentioned in the "Eight Ways to Punch Up P.M. Meals" (page 96), keep these basics on hand:

▶ Your favorite frozen fruits and vegetables—the fruits for a quick fruit salad, the veggies for sautés and stir-fries
▶ Frozen chicken and turkey (boneless, skinless pieces are healthiest and quickest)
▶ Frozen fish fillets (not breaded), shrimp, or scallops
▶ Canned tuna or salmon in oil or water
▶ Tofu—firm or extra-firm for stir-fries

SET ASIDE ONE HOUR OF PREP TIME PER WEEK. As soon as you get home from the grocery store, start prepping. Portion large containers of cottage cheese and yogurt into single-size servings; cook and divide large cuts of meat, poultry, or fish into 3-ounce portions; wash, peel, and slice any fruits, vegetables, and salad greens you have for the week.

CHEAT WITH PREPPED PRODUCE. Eating a lot of fruits and veggies doesn't have to mean a lot of slicing, dicing, and chopping. Opt for prewashed and peeled veggies (salad greens and spinach, baby carrots, grape tomatoes, chopped cauliflower and broccoli). They're cleaned, cut, and ready to go. If you want fruit salad, hit the salad bar at the supermarket for melon, berries, and pineapple. Many convenience stores offer fruit salad as well.

PICK UP A ROTISSERIE CHICKEN. Available in large supermarkets, these juicy, ready-to-eat birds can be eaten as is or sliced for salads and stir-fries.

COOK FISH FAST. Try preparing fish *en papilotte* (French for little paper packages), with parchment paper or foil. Instructions can be found online—you can cook fish in as little as 15 minutes.

MAKE ENOUGH DINNER FOR TOMORROW'S LUNCH. If you're responsible for your family's dinner, grill extra fish, poultry, or chicken for your midday meal. Prepare an extra serving of roasted, grilled, or sautéed vegetables, too. If, however, being in the kitchen at that hour threatens to derail your diet with temptation, steer clear.

6

THE
PLAN

ow you understand how eating in sync with your body's
natural rhythms controls your hunger and breaks your
addiction to sweets and starches, which helps you
achieve the fit body you've always wanted. But before
you begin my program, close your eyes for a moment. Imagine
yourself four short weeks from now.

You're pounds lighter and halfway through your daily walk.
Your pace is brisk—you slept well, so your mood is bright and
your energy is off the charts. Your waist is inches slimmer; your
muscles are more toned; your skin glows with health. A stressful
day no longer drives you to a pint of rocky road ice cream. Best
of all, you're eating the foods you love—and still losing weight.

That's a motivating image, isn't it? The best part is, it
doesn't have to remain a vision. With the help of the three meal
formulas (found together on page 172), the Big Breakfast Diet
plan leads you day by day, meal by delicious meal toward that
fitter, healthier you. Now that you have my specific guidelines on
what to eat and *when,* you can expect to:

THE SKINNY

Apply the breakfast, lunch, and dinner formulas to your pantry to build satisfying meals and put the Big Breakfast Diet into action. Follow the diet and record your progress to keep the weight coming off.

▶ rev up your metabolism,

▶ burn more calories by day and more fat at night,

▶ enjoy your favorite foods as you lose weight,

▶ satisfy your hunger all day,

▶ eliminate cravings for sweets and starches,

▶ feel alert and refreshed when you awaken in the morning, rather than sluggish and foggy,

▶ enjoy energy to burn, and

▶ reduce your risk for serious health conditions such as type 2 diabetes and heart disease.

How the Plan Works

Each day of the Big Breakfast Diet program you will build meals using the Formulas (page 172) and the Servings List (page 54). At the start, record your progress in "The First 28 Days," a fill-in workbook beginning on page 173. Divided into sections (The Menu, The Workout, and The Cure for Cravings), here's what you'll find.

The pages that follow contain your daily menu options—specifically, they include ten tasty breakfasts, seven lunches, and seven dinners, plus six vegetarian or vegan meals. Try each meal, stick with a few favorites, or make your own using the formulas; it's your choice. Make sure you jot down what you chose for each meal in "The First 28 Days" so you can remember what you liked and didn't like, and what meals satisfied your hunger best.

The Menu section gives you the opportunity to reflect on your personal food-related "news." Which meal did you enjoy most, and why? Did you find it a challenge to plan or eat your breakfast?

How might you solve those issues tomorrow? Did you get hungry at night? If so, did you eat enough protein at breakfast? In what way can you increase your protein servings at breakfast?

You can also use the fill-in section to explore how eating in sync affects your hunger and appetite. Do you feel less hungry or experience fewer cravings? Did a stressful day trigger cravings for sugar or starches, even though you weren't hungry? Were you able to stick to the plan?

The Workout section of the plan (explained in chapter 8) contains your daily workout—your choice of a walk or one or more 10-Minute Workouts. In week one, you'll start with a 20-minute walk or one or two of the workouts. By week four, you may be able to walk forty minutes or perform three or four 10-Minute Workouts.

The fill-in section under Workout in "The First 28 Days" invites you to reflect on your physical activity. Jot down your observations every day about that day's walk or workout. What did you enjoy about it? What was a challenge? Were you energized or fatigued?

The Cure for Cravings is a daily tip to help you manage cravings and other food temptations. It's all part of sticking to your workout, reducing stress, and getting a restful night's sleep (so you can burn more fat). Not every tip will work for you, but you're sure to find plenty that will help you master your hunger, cravings, and weight.

As you follow this program, write daily entries in the fill-in areas provided. Don't panic—no need to write pages and pages. A line or two in each section will help you explore your relationship with food, identify your personal eating behaviors and "hot button" issues that tend to derail—or enhance—your weight-loss success.

Don't forget your vision of yourself, either. Close your eyes and revisit that fitter, slimmer you each morning. Stick to the Big Breakfast Diet plan and just 28 days from today you'll have turned that vision into reality.

30 Mix-and-Match Big Breakfast
MEAL PLANS
WITH RECIPES

Before you begin the Big Breakfast plan, take a look at some of the delicious meals you'll enjoy for the next four weeks. Choose one breakfast, one lunch, and one dinner every day, or better yet, build your own using the formulas. Mix and match them as you like. Feel free to sample all 30 meals, or just stick with your favorites or just use them as inspiration when you concoct your own. The only rules: Eat at least seven servings of protein in the morning, and always eat your breakfast sweet.

You can combine Breakfast 1 with Lunch 5 and with Dinner 7 to eat well and be satisfied all day. Or take Breakfast 5, Lunch 2, and Dinner 1—the idea is to inspire you with options and give you the freedom to choose what you want to eat. If you like more "breakfast-y" foods for breakfast, go for the French toast in Breakfast 5; if you like to eat your family's dinner leftovers, try the pizza (Breakfast 7).

Each recipe represents a single serving size, so multiply accordingly if you're cooking for more than one. Build your plan in the pages of "The First 28 Days" starting on page 173 and be sure to take notes in the journal so you can keep track of particular meals and recipes that work well for you.

If you're especially short on time, choose one of the Dine-and-Dash meals marked with a 🏹. Those meals are noted as being particularly easy to prepare or easy to transport (it's much easier to take a turkey sandwich to go than it is an egg scramble!).

Remember that, ultimately, the formulas rule. Use them as your guide and your meal options become infinite.

10 Breakfast Meal Plans
WITH RECIPES

These meals are only suggestions of what you can eat on the Big Breakfast Diet. Let the variety of meals in the pages ahead inspire you—once you understand how the formulas work (see page 172), let them be your guide.

GETTING YOUR
MILK PROTEIN

In the Breakfast Formula on page 75, it explains that two of your morning proteins must be milk- or yogurt-based—but you still have choices as to how you consume them!

OPTION 1: LOW-FAT MILK
2 protein servings = 16 ounces milk

OPTION 2: THE SHAKE
2 protein servings = 8 ounces low-fat milk or soy milk and 3 tablespoons of whey

OPTION 3: THE SMOOTHIE
2 protein servings = 8 ounces plain, low-fat yogurt and 3 tablespoons of whey

BREAKFAST 1

✳ **The Shake, The Smoothie,** *or* 16 ounces of low-fat milk
See page 50 for recipes.

✳ **Country-Style Egg White Scramble**

Cooking oil spray
3 egg whites (1 serving)
2 ounces (2 servings) cheddar cheese, torn or shredded
2 ounces (2 servings) lean ham, chopped
1 medium-size tomato (optional), diced
½ medium-size onion (optional), diced

Spray a small nonstick skillet with cooking oil spray. Heat the
skillet over medium heat. Add the egg whites, cheese, ham,
and tomato and/or onion, if desired. Cook, stirring, until the
eggs are cooked through to taste.

✳ **Cereal**

1 serving cereal of your choice (see page 59)
8 ounces low-fat milk or soy milk

✳ **Toast**

½ English muffin
2 tablespoons cream cheese or 1 tablespoon peanut butter

Toast the English muffin half and spread it with the cream
cheese or peanut butter.

✳ **Breakfast Sweet**

1 serving, see page 69.

PROTEINS 7 SERVINGS	2 servings of low-fat or soy milk or yogurt	The Shake, The Smoothie, or 16 ounces of low-fat milk
	1 serving of eggs	3 egg whites: Country-Style Egg White Scramble
	2 servings of cheese	2 ounces of cheddar: Country-Style Egg White Scramble
	2 servings of meat, chicken, or fish	2 ounces of ham: Country-Style Egg White Scramble

CARBOHYDRATES 3 SERVINGS	2 servings of bread or starches	½ of an English muffin and ½ cup of cereal
	1 serving	A breakfast sweet
FATS 2 SERVINGS		2 tablespoons of cream cheese or 1 tablespoon of peanut butter

BREAKFAST 2

* **The Shake, The Smoothie,** *or* 16 ounces of low-fat milk
  See page 50 for recipes.

* **Turkey and Cheese Sandwich**

  2 slices bread

  2 tablespoons reduced-fat mayonnaise

  3 ounces (6 slices; 3 servings) smoked turkey

  2 ounces (4 slices; 2 servings) Swiss cheese

  Lettuce, tomato, and/or mustard (optional)

  Salt and freshly ground black pepper (optional)

  Toast the bread, then spread it with the mayonnaise. Top one slice of bread with the turkey and cheese. Add lettuce, tomato, and/or mustard and season with salt and pepper, if desired. Sandwich with the second slice of bread.

* **Breakfast Sweet**

  1 serving, see page 69.

PROTEINS 7 SERVINGS	2 servings of low-fat or soy milk or yogurt	The Shake, The Smoothie, or 16 ounces of low-fat milk
	2 servings of cheese	2 ounces of Swiss cheese: Turkey and Cheese Sandwich
	3 servings of meat, chicken, or fish	3 ounces of turkey: Turkey and Cheese Sandwich
CARBOHYDRATES 3 SERVINGS	2 servings of bread or starches	2 slices of bread: Turkey and Cheese Sandwich
	1 serving	A breakfast sweet
FATS 2 SERVINGS		2 tablespoons of reduced-fat mayonnaise: Turkey and Cheese Sandwich

✈ BREAKFAST 3

❋ **The Shake, The Smoothie,** *or* 16 ounces of low-fat milk
See page 50 for recipes.

❋ **Smoked Salmon Bagel**

> 1 small bagel, cut in half
> 2 tablespoons (2 servings) cream cheese
> 4 to 5 ounces (4 to 5 servings) smoked salmon
> ⅓ cup thinly sliced red onion (optional)
> Freshly ground black pepper
> 2 lemon wedges (optional), for garnish

Toast the bagel, then spread each half with the cream cheese.
Top with the smoked salmon and onion, if desired. Season
with pepper to taste. Garnish with lemon, if desired.

❋ **Breakfast Sweet**

> 1 serving, see page 69.

PROTEINS 7 SERVINGS	2 servings of low-fat or soy milk or yogurt	The Shake, The Smoothie, or 16 ounces of low-fat milk
	5 servings of meat, chicken, or fish	4 to 5 ounces smoked salmon
CARBOHYDRATES 3 SERVINGS	2 servings of bread or starches	1 small bagel
	1 serving	A breakfast sweet
FATS 2 SERVINGS	2 servings	2 tablespoons of cream cheese

✈ BREAKFAST 4

❋ **The Shake, The Smoothie,** *or* 16 ounces of low-fat milk
See page 50 for recipes.

❋ **Fish Tacos**

> ¾ cup (1 serving) plain low-fat yogurt
> 2 tablepsoons (2 servings) reduced-fat mayonnaise

Juice of 1 lime

½ teaspoon dried oregano

½ teaspoon ground cumin

Salt and freshly ground black pepper

Cooking oil spray

4 ounces (4 servings) fish fillet of your choice,
  such as sole or flounder

4 taco shells (2 servings)

1 cup shredded cabbage

1 medium-size tomato, diced

1 jalapeño pepper (optional), minced

Place the yogurt, mayonnaise, and lime juice in a small bowl and stir to mix. Add the oregano and cumin. Season with salt and pepper to taste. Set the dressing aside.

Spray a nonstick skillet with cooking oil spray. Add the fish fillet and cook over medium-high heat until the fish turns opaque and flakes when pierced with a fork, 3 to 4 minutes per side. Chop the fish and divide it equally among the 4 taco shells. Spoon equal portions of the dressing over each taco. Top each taco with cabbage, tomato, and jalapeño, if desired.

✳ Breakfast Sweet

1 serving, see page 69.

PROTEINS 7 SERVINGS	3 servings of low-fat or soy milk or yogurt	The Shake, The Smoothie or 16 ounces of low-fat milk and ¾ cup low-fat yogurt: Fish Tacos
	4 servings of meat, chicken, or fish	4 ounces of fish fillet: Fish Tacos
CARBOHYDRATES 3 SERVINGS	2 servings of bread or starches	4 taco shells: Fish Tacos
	1 serving	A breakfast sweet
FATS 2 SERVINGS		2 tablespoons of reduced-fat mayonnaise: Fish Tacos

BREAKFAST 5

* **The Shake, The Smoothie,** *or* 16 ounces of low-fat milk
See page 50 for recipes.

* **French Toast with Whipped YoBerry Topping**

FOR THE WHIPPED YOBERRY TOPPING

1 cup frozen or thawed berries

¾ cup (1 serving) plain low-fat yogurt

Splenda or other sugar substitute

FOR THE FRENCH TOAST

Cooking oil spray

3 egg whites

2 tablespoons low-fat milk

½ teaspoon ground cinnamon

¼ teaspoon vanilla extract

2 slices whole-grain bread

2 teaspoons (2 servings) butter

Fresh mint leaves, for garnish (optional)

Make the Whipped YoBerry Topping: Set aside a few whole berries for topping the French toast. Place the remaining berries and the yogurt in a blender and blend on high speed until creamy, about 30 seconds. Add sugar substitute to taste, then set the topping aside.

Make the French toast: Spray a nonstick skillet with cooking oil spray. Place the egg whites, low-fat milk, cinnamon, and vanilla extract in a large, shallow bowl and stir to mix. Soak one slice of bread until saturated, turning to coat both sides. Melt 1 teaspoon of the butter in the prepared skillet over medium-high heat. Cook the soaked slice of bread, turning it once, until each side is lightly browned. Transfer the slice of French toast to a plate and cover it to keep warm. Repeat with the remaining slice of bread and 1 teaspoon of butter. Spread the whipped topping on the French toast and top it with the reserved berries and a mint garnish, if desired.

✴ Protein of Your Choice
3 servings

Breakfast Sweet
The Whipped YoBerry Topping takes the place of the breakfast sweet here.

PROTEINS 7 SERVINGS	2 servings of low-fat or soy milk or yogurt	The Shake, The Smoothie, or 16 ounces of low-fat milk
	2 servings	Contained in the French Toast with Whipped YoBerry Topping
	3 servings of meat, chicken, or fish	3 links of turkey sausage
CARBOHYDRATES 3 SERVINGS	2 servings bread or starches	Contained in the French Toast
	1 serving	Contained in the Whipped YoBerry Topping
FATS 2 SERVINGS		2 teaspoons of butter in the French Toast

↗ BREAKFAST 6

✴ The Shake, The Smoothie, *or* 16 ounces of low-fat milk
See page 50 for recipes.

✴ Tuna Melt

3 ounces (3 servings) water-packed canned tuna, drained

¼ cup sliced pickles (optional)

2 tablespoons (2 servings) reduced-fat mayonnaise

1 tablespoon ketchup

2 teaspoons mustard

2 slices (2 servings) rye bread

2 ounces (4 slices; 2 servings) Swiss cheese

1 medium-size tomato, sliced

Salt and freshly ground black pepper

Chopped chives, for garnish (optional)

➡

Preheat the oven to 350°F. Place the tuna, pickles, if desired, and the mayonnaise, ketchup, and mustard in a bowl and stir to mix. Spread the tuna mixture on top of one slice of rye bread. Top with the Swiss cheese and tomato. Season with salt and pepper to taste, then sandwich with the second slice of rye bread. Toast the sandwich in the oven until the cheese melts, 5 to 10 minutes. Garnish with chives, if desired.

✳ Breakfast Sweet
1 serving, see page 69.

PROTEINS 7 SERVINGS	2 servings of low-fat or soy milk or yogurt	The Shake, The Smoothie, or 16 ounces of low-fat milk
	2 servings of cheese	2 ounces of Swiss cheese: Tuna Melt
	3 servings of meat, chicken, or fish	3 ounces of canned tuna: Tuna Melt
CARBOHYDRATES 3 SERVINGS	2 servings of bread or starches	2 slices of rye bread: Tuna Melt
	1 serving	A breakfast sweet
FATS 2 SERVINGS		2 tablespoons of reduced-fat mayonnaise: Tuna Melt

BREAKFAST 7

✳ The Shake, The Smoothie, or 16 ounces of low-fat milk
See page 50 for recipes.

✳ Pizza in the Morning
1 slice thin-crust store-bought pizza (one half of a 12-inch pie)

Top the pizza with 3 ounces of sliced pepperoni and reheat it. If you have some fresh basil, add it as well.

OR MAKE YOUR OWN
2 teaspoons olive oil
One 6-inch pita
2 ounces (4 slices; 2 servings) mozzarella cheese

1 small tomato, thinly sliced

½ small onion (optional), thinly sliced

3 ounces (3 servings) turkey pepperoni

Chopped fresh basil

Salt and freshly ground black pepper

Preheat the oven to 450°F. Brush the olive oil on one side of the pita and place it on a baking sheet, oiled side up. Top the pita with the mozzarella, tomato, onion, if desired, and turkey pepperoni. Sprinkle some basil on top and season with salt and pepper to taste. Bake the pizza until the cheese melts, about 5 minutes.

✳ Breakfast Sweet

1 serving, see page 69.

PROTEINS 7 SERVINGS	2 servings of low-fat or soy milk or yogurt	The Shake, The Smoothie, or 16 ounces of low-fat milk
	5 servings	Contained in the Pizza in the Morning
CARBOHYDRATES 3 SERVINGS	2 servings of bread or starches	Crust of Pizza in the Morning
	1 serving	A breakfast sweet
FATS 2 SERVINGS		Contained in the Pizza in the Morning

BREAKFAST 8

✳ The Shake, The Smoothie, *or* 16 ounces of low-fat milk

See page 50 for recipes.

✳ Pancakes with Very Berry Syrup

FOR THE BERRY SYRUP

½ cup fresh or frozen berries

1 teaspoon vanilla extract

2 teaspoons Splenda or other sugar substitute,
   or more if necessary

FOR THE PANCAKES

¾ cup all-purpose flour

1 teaspoon baking powder

¼ teaspoon salt

1 teaspoon Splenda or other sugar substitute

¼ cup and 1 tablespoon milk (no need to count this milk serving
toward your protein servings)

1 egg (1 serving)

Cooking oil spray

2 teaspoons butter

½ cup (1 serving) low-fat ricotta

Make the berry syrup: Set aside a few whole berries for topping
the pancakes. Place the remaining berries in a deep bowl
and crush them with a potato masher. Transfer the mashed
berries to a small saucepan and cook over low heat until
warmed through, about 5 minutes. Add the vanilla extract
and sugar substitute. Taste for sweetness, adding more sugar
substitute, if desired. Set the berry syrup aside.

Make the pancakes: Place the flour, baking powder, salt, and
sugar substitute in a bowl and stir to mix. Make a well in
the center, add the milk and egg, and stir to mix. Spray a
griddle or nonstick skillet with cooking oil spray. Add the
butter and heat over medium-high heat. Using a ladle, pour
scoops of the batter onto the hot griddle or skillet to form
approximately 6-inch pancakes. When bubbles begin to
form in the pancakes turn them and cook until the second
side is browned, about 1 minute longer. Transfer the
pancakes to a plate, top them with the ricotta, and pour
the berry syrup over them. Garnish the pancakes with the
reserved berries.

NOTE: You may use a sugar-free pancake syrup, sweetened with
Splenda or other sugar substitute, in place of the berry syrup.

✳ **Protein of Your Choice**

3 servings

⁕ **Breakfast Sweet**
1 serving, see page 69.

PROTEINS 7 SERVINGS	2 servings of low-fat or soy milk or yogurt	The Shake, The Smoothie, or 16 ounces of low-fat milk
	2 servings	Contained in the pancakes
	3 servings of meat, chicken, or fish	3 slices of Canadian bacon
CARBOHYDRATES 3 SERVINGS	2 servings of bread or starches	Contained in the Pancakes with Very Berry Syrup
	1 serving	A breakfast sweet
FATS 2 SERVINGS		2 teaspoons of butter in the pancakes

BREAKFAST 9

⁕ **The Shake, The Smoothie,** *or* 16 ounces of low-fat milk
See page 50 for recipes.

⁕ **Cowpoke Breakfast Steak**

2 tablespoons (1 serving) grated Parmesan cheese

1 tablespoon ketchup

2 tablespoons (2 servings) reduced-fat mayonnaise

Cooking oil spray

4 ounces (4 servings) lean beef steak of your choice

Salt and freshly ground black pepper

2 slices of French or Italian bread (½ inch thick)

Put the Parmesan, ketchup, and mayonnaise in a small bowl and stir to mix. Preheat the broiler and spray a broiler pan with cooking oil spray; or spray a nonstick skillet with cooking oil spray and heat it over medium-high heat. Place the steak in the broiler pan or skillet and cook until done to taste. To test for doneness, insert an instant-read meat thermometer in the center of the steak; when it is done to medium-rare the thermometer will register 145°F.

Season the steak with salt and pepper to taste, top it with the Parmesan and ketchup sauce, and serve the bread on the side.

✷ Breakfast Sweet
1 serving, see page 69.

PROTEINS 7 SERVINGS	2 servings of low-fat milk or yogurt	The Shake, The Smoothie, or 16 ounces of low-fat milk
	1 serving of cheese	2 tablespoons of Parmesan cheese: Cowpoke Breakfast Steak
	4 servings of meat, chicken, or fish	4 ounces of beef steak: Cowpoke Breakfast Steak
CARBOHYDRATES 3 SERVINGS	2 servings of bread or starches	2 slices of French or Italian bread
	1 serving	A breakfast sweet
FATS 2 SERVINGS		2 tablespoons of reduced-fat mayonnaise: Cowpoke Breakfast Steak

BREAKFAST 10

✷ The Shake, The Smoothie, *or* 16 ounces of low-fat milk
See page 50 for recipes.

✷ Chicken Breakfast Burrito
  Cooking oil spray
  2 teaspoons (2 servings) butter
  2 cups (2 servings) sliced mushrooms
  3 ounces (3 servings) precooked chicken breast, diced
  Salt and freshly ground black pepper
  Chopped fresh flat-leaf parsley
  2 ounces (2 servings) Monterey Jack cheese, torn or shredded
  1 large (8 inch) whole-wheat tortilla
  2 tablespoons fresh tomato salsa

Spray a small nonstick skillet with cooking oil spray. Add the butter and heat over medium heat. Add the mushrooms and cook, stirring, until browned. Add the chicken and cook, stirring, until warmed through. Season with salt, pepper, and parsley to taste. Stir in the cheese. Place the tortilla on a work surface and spoon the chicken mixture over it. Roll up the tortilla like a burrito and garnish with the salsa.

*Breakfast Sweet
1 serving, see page 69.

PROTEINS	2 servings of low-fat or soy milk or yogurt	The Shake, The Smoothie, or 16 ounces of low-fat milk
7 SERVINGS		
	2 servings of cheese	2 ounces of Monterey Jack cheese: Chicken Breakfast Burrito
	3 servings of meat, chicken, or fish	3 ounces of chicken: Chicken Breakfast Burrito
CARBOHYDRATES 3 SERVINGS	2 servings bread or starches	1 large whole wheat tortilla: Chicken Breakfast Burrito
	1 serving	A breakfast sweet
FATS 2 SERVINGS		2 teaspoons of butter: Chicken Breakfast Burrito

7 Lunch Meal Plans
WITH RECIPES

Lunches should be satisfying. As you build your meal or peruse a menu during your lunch break, make sure you satisfy the required protein serving. Whether you're at home and have time to prepare lunch or you're going out to eat with colleagues, dishes like the ones here will inspire you to follow the lunch formula with ease. Take note of how you feel on the first few days on the diet; if you're hungry before lunch, don't modify your lunch plan, simply add more protein to your breakfast the following day. Never change your lunch formula! Just keep challenging yourself to come up with tasty variations. Note: If you're short on time, choose one of the Dine-and-Dash meals marked with an arrow ($\nearrow$).

LUNCH 1

✳ Hearty Chef's Special

> 3 servings (3 ounces) of the meat, chicken,
> or fish protein of your choice
> 3 servings your choice of vegetables from Vegetable Group A
> (see page 66)
> 2 servings your choice of vegetables from Vegetable Group B
> (see page 67)
> Salad dressing of your choice, preferably no-sugar and fat-free

Combine the protein in a large bowl with the vegetables from Group A and Group B. Top with the salad dressing.

✳ Fruit

1 serving, see pages 67–68.

LUNCH 2

✳ Fish in a Packet

> 3 ounces (3 servings) fresh or thawed frozen fish fillet
> ½ lemon, thinly sliced
> 1 teaspoon olive oil
> 1 sprig fresh basil or parsley, chopped
> Salt and freshly ground black pepper

Preheat the oven to 350°F. Place the fish in the center of a square of heavy-duty aluminum foil. Top the fish with the lemon, olive oil, and basil or parsley, then season it with salt and pepper to taste. Pull the aluminum foil up over the fish and loosely fold the edges together to seal the packet. Place the packet on a baking sheet and bake the fish until it is opaque, 12 to 15 minutes. To test for doneness, open the packet and pierce the fish with a fork; it should break into flakes. Place the opened packet on a plate for serving.

✳ Sliced Tomato, Cucumber, and Onion Salad

> 2 medium-size tomatoes (2 servings)
> 1 cup thinly sliced peeled cucumber (1 serving)

Thinly sliced sweet white or red onion (from 1 serving)

2 tablespoons balsamic vinegar

1 tablespoon lemon juice

1 tablespoon olive oil

1 sprig fresh basil, chopped

1 sprig fresh parsley, chopped

Salt and freshly ground black pepper

Core and thinly slice the tomatoes. Arrange the tomatoes, cucumber, and onion on a large plate. Place the balsamic vinegar, lemon juice, and olive oil in a small bowl and whisk until well blended. Brush the dressing over the vegetables and sprinkle the basil and parsley on top. Season the salad with salt and pepper to taste.

❋ Vegetables

2 servings of vegetables from Vegetable Group B, see page 67.

❋ Fruit

1 serving, see pages 67–68.

LUNCH 3

❋ Turkey or Chicken Salad

FOR THE SALAD DRESSING

2 to 3 tablespoons plain nonfat yogurt

1 teaspoon fat-free mayonnaise

¾ teaspoon fresh lemon juice

1 tablespoon chopped fresh basil, or

⅓ teaspoon dried basil

¼ teaspoon dried thyme

¼ teaspoon freshly ground black pepper

FOR THE TURKEY OR CHICKEN SALAD

¼ small red onion

1 stalk celery

½ small apple (½ serving)

6 grapes (½ serving)

3 ounces (3 servings) chopped cooked turkey or
chicken breast

2 red bell peppers or 2 tomatoes

1 tablespoon fresh parsley

¼ teaspoon paprika

Make the salad dressing: Place the yogurt, mayonnaise, lemon juice, basil, thyme, and black pepper in a small bowl and whisk until well blended. Set the salad dressing aside.

Make the salad: Chop the red onion, celery, and apple and place them in a medium-size bowl. Cut the grapes in half and add them to the bowl. Add the turkey or chicken and the salad dressing and toss until well mixed. Cut the bell peppers or tomatoes in half. Trim and seed the bell peppers or core the tomatoes. Arrange the bell peppers or tomatoes on a plate. Stuff the bell peppers or tomatoes with the salad and sprinkle the parsley and paprika on top.

⚹ Vegetables

2 servings of vegetables from Vegetable Group B, see page 67.

LUNCH 4

⚹ Broiled Salmon with Cilantro-Mint Dressing

2 tablespoons plain low-fat yogurt

1 teaspoon minced fresh cilantro

½ teaspoon chopped fresh mint

¼ small cucumber, peeled, seeded, and finely chopped

Salt and freshly ground black pepper

Cooking oil spray

3 ounces (3 servings) salmon or other fish fillet

1 teaspoon olive oil

Place the yogurt, cilantro, mint, and cucumber in a small bowl and stir to mix. Season the dressing with salt and pepper to taste, then set the dressing aside. Preheat the broiler. Spray a broiler pan with cooking oil spray. Brush the fish fillet with the olive oil, place the fish in the prepared broiler pan, and broil until the top side is golden, about 5 minutes. Turn the fish over and broil it until it is opaque but juicy and flakes when pierced with a fork, 3 to 4 minutes longer. Top the fish with the cilantro-mint dressing.

✳ Vegetables

3 servings of vegetables from Vegetable Group A and 2 servings of vegetables from Vegetable Group B, see pages 66–67.

✳ Fruit

1 serving, see pages 67–68.

LUNCH 5

✳ Zesty Flank Steak with Roasted Asparagus

> 3 ounces (3 servings) flank steak
>
> 1 tablespoon fresh lemon juice
>
> 1 tablespoon soy sauce
>
> ¼ teaspoon minced garlic
>
> ¼ teaspoon grated peeled fresh ginger
>
> ¼ teaspoon chopped jalapeño pepper
>
> (wear plastic gloves to protect your skin when chopping)
>
> ¼ bunch of asparagus, tough ends removed
>
> ¼ tablespoon extra-virgin olive oil
>
> Salt and freshly ground pepper

Combine the flank steak, lemon juice, soy sauce, garlic, ginger, and jalapeño pepper in a large resealable plastic bag and shake until the flank steak is thoroughly coated. Let the flank steak marinate in the refrigerator for 30 minutes, turning it occasionally.

Preheat the oven to 400°F. Toss the asparagus with the olive oil and season it with salt and black pepper to taste. Arrange the asparagus in a single layer on a rimmed baking sheet and bake it until soft and lightly brown, about 10 minutes. Set the roasted asparagus aside.

Preheat the grill to high. Drain the flank steak, setting aside the marinade. Grill the steak until done to taste, basting it frequently with the reserved marinade but not during the last minutes of grilling on either side. To test for doneness, insert an instant-read meat thermometer in the center of the steak; when it is done to medium-rare the thermometer will register 145°F. Cut the flank steak into thin slices on a diagonal across the grain and serve with the asparagus.

✳ Vegetables

2 servings each of vegetables from Vegetable Group A and Vegetable Group B, see pages 66–67.

✳ Fruit

1 serving, see pages 67–68.

LUNCH 6

✳ Parmesan Chicken Fingers

Cooking oil spray

3 ounces (3 servings) skinless, boneless chicken breast, cut into 1-inch strips

2 tablespoons fat-free milk

2 tablespoons seasoned dried bread crumbs

1 tablespoon grated Parmesan cheese

1 sprig fresh parsley, chopped

¼ teaspoon freshly ground black pepper

2 tablespoons low-calorie honey-mustard dressing (optional)

Preheat the oven to 400°F. Spray a baking sheet with cooking oil spray. Place the chicken in a shallow bowl and pierce it with a fork. Add the milk, stir to mix, and refrigerate the chicken, covered, for 15 minutes. Combine the bread crumbs, Parmesan cheese, parsley, and pepper in another shallow bowl. Drain the chicken and dip it into the bread crumb mixture, turning to coat well. Bake the chicken on the prepared baking sheet until cooked through, about 10 minutes per side, then serve with the honey-mustard dressing, if desired.

✳ Vegetables

3 servings of vegetables from Vegetable Group A and 2 servings from Vegetable Group B, see pages 66–67.

- -

LUNCH 7

Lemon-Lime Scallops

> 2 teaspoons olive oil
> Up to 3 ounces (up to 3 servings) sea scallops,
>   rinsed, dried, and quartered
> 1 tablespoon fat-free margarine
> ¼ clove garlic, minced
> 1 sprig fresh parsley, minced
> ¼ teaspoon paprika
> Fresh lemon and/or lime juice
>   (juice of ½ to 1 small fruit)
> Salt and freshly ground black pepper

Heat the olive oil in a saucepan over medium-high heat. Add the scallops and cook, stirring frequently, until just golden brown, 6 to 8 minutes. Transfer the scallops to a serving plate and loosely cover them with aluminum foil to keep warm. Add the margarine, garlic, parsley, paprika, and lemon and/or lime juice to the same saucepan and cook until the margarine melts. Season the sauce with salt and pepper to taste, then pour over the scallops.

✳ Vegetables

3 servings of vegetables from Vegetable Group A and 2 servings from Vegetable Group B, see pages 66–67.

✳ Fruit

1 serving, see pages 67–68.

7 Dinner Meal Plans
WITH RECIPES

After lunch, you may want to enjoy a light dinner. Once the diet begins to kick in you'll probably find you can skip dinner altogether. Though social engagements around dinnertime may pose a challenge at first, you'll come to realize that your breakfast and lunch meals have prepared you well. That said, if you feel the need to snack between lunch and dinner, enjoy any of the vegetables in Vegetable Group A, or keep a container of The Stew (see page 52) on hand. And, if you like, you may round out any of the dinner main courses with some of The Stew in place of the veggies from Group A. Be sure to track your cravings in the fill-in sections of "The First 28 Days" so you can adjust your diet appropriately. Note: If you're short on time, choose the Dine-and-Dash meal marked with an arrow (✈).

DINNER 1

✱ Goat Cheese and Baby Spinach Salad

FOR THE SALAD DRESSING

3 tablespoons balsamic vinegar

1 tablespoon olive oil

Salt and freshly ground black pepper

FOR THE SALAD

1 to 2 cups (1 to 2 servings) baby spinach

1 to 2 servings your choice of vegetables from Vegetable Group A
(see page 66)

2 servings your choice of vegetables from Vegetable Group B
(see page 67)

Up to 3 ounces (up to 3 servings) low-fat or fat-free goat cheese
or another cheese of your choice (see page 54)

Make the salad dressing: Place the balsamic vinegar and olive oil in a small bowl and whisk until well blended. Season the salad dressing with salt and pepper to taste.

Make the salad: Rinse and dry the baby spinach, then tear it into bite-size pieces. Place the spinach in a large bowl and add the vegetables from Groups A and B. Pour the dressing over the salad and toss to mix. Top the salad with the cheese (goat cheese crumbles are nice with this salad).

✳ Fruit

1 serving each of fruit from Group A and Group B, see pages 67–68.

DINNER 2

Spicy Thai Beef

FOR THE STEAK

Cooking oil spray

3 ounces (3 servings) trimmed boneless beef
   top round steak

FOR THE SALAD

1 teaspoon fresh lime juice

1 teaspoon Asian fish sauce

1 teaspoon olive oil

1 teaspoon chopped garlic

Crushed red pepper flakes

1 to 2 cups (1 to 2 servings) greens of your choice
   (see page 67)

1 to 2 servings your choice of vegetables from Vegetable Group A
   (see page 66)

2 servings your choice of vegetables from Vegetable Group B
   (see page 67)

1 sprig fresh cilantro, coarsely chopped

1 sprig fresh mint, coarsely chopped

Salt and freshly ground black pepper

Prepare the steak: Spray a nonstick skillet with cooking oil spray and heat it over medium-high heat. Add the steak and cook until done to taste. Use an instant-read meat thermometer inserted in the center of the steak to test for doneness; medium-rare steak will register 145°F on the thermometer. Transfer the cooked steak to a plate and set it aside.

Make the salad: Place the lime juice, fish sauce, olive oil, and garlic in a large bowl and whisk until well blended. Season with red pepper flakes to taste. Add the greens, the vegetables from Groups A and B, and the cilantro and mint and toss until well mixed. Season the salad with salt and black pepper to taste. Cut the steak on a diagonal into thin slices and arrange these on top of the salad. Drizzle the juices from the steak on top.

✳ Fruit

2 servings each of fruit from Group A and Group B, see pages 67–68.

DINNER 3

✳ Sliced Cheese

Up to 3 servings of the cheese of your choice (see page 54); a soft cheese, such as Brie, is nice.

✳ Fruit Salad

> 1 serving each of the fruit of your choice from Group A and Group B (see pages 67–68)
>
> ¼ cup fresh lime juice
>
> 2 fresh mint sprigs (optional), chopped
>
> Splenda or other sugar substitute

Rinse, slice, and chop the fruit, then place it in a bowl. Place the lime juice, mint, if using, and a pinch of sugar substitute in a small bowl and stir to mix. Pour the lime juice mixture over the fruit and gently toss until coated.

✳ Vegetables

At least 3 servings of vegetables from Vegetable Group A and 2 servings from Vegetable Group B, see pages 66–67.

DINNER 4

✳ Sautéed Shrimp and Peppery Red Cabbage

FOR THE SALAD

1 tablespoon olive oil

1 teaspoon apple cider vinegar

¼ teaspoon Dijon mustard

¼ teaspoon crushed red pepper flakes

Salt and freshly ground black pepper

1 cup (1 serving) shredded red cabbage

1 large carrot, grated

FOR THE SHRIMP AND VEGETABLES

Cooking oil spray

Up to 6 ounces (up to 3 servings) large shrimp,
    peeled and deveined

2 servings each your choice of vegetables from Vegetable Group A
    and Vegetable Group B (see pages 66–67)

Make the salad: Place the olive oil, cider vinegar, mustard, and red pepper flakes in a large bowl and whisk until well blended. Season with salt and black pepper to taste. Add the red cabbage and carrot and toss until well mixed. Set the salad aside.

Prepare the shrimp: Spray a nonstick skillet with cooking oil spray and heat it over medium heat. Add the shrimp and cook them until firm and opaque, about 8 minutes. Serve the shrimp over the salad along with the vegetables from Vegetable Group A and/or B.

✳ Fruit

1 serving each of fruit from Group A and Group B, see pages 67–68.

DINNER 5

✳ Niçoise Salad

FOR THE SALAD DRESSING

1 tablespoon lemon juice

1 tablespoon olive oil

1 tablespoon minced fresh thyme

1 sprig fresh basil, chopped, or dried basil to taste

1 sprig fresh oregano, chopped, or dried oregano to taste

½ teaspoon Dijon mustard

Salt and freshly ground black pepper

FOR THE SALAD

At least 2 cups (2 servings) greens of your choice (see page 67)

Up to 3 ounces grilled tuna, or 1½ cups (up to 3 ounces) drained
   canned water-packed tuna (3 servings)

1 medium-size tomato (1 serving)

1 cup steamed string beans (2 servings)

Thinly sliced red onion (from 1 serving)

Salt and freshly ground black pepper

2 tablespoons capers (optional)

Make the salad dressing: Place the lemon juice, olive oil,
thyme, basil, oregano, and mustard in a small bowl and whisk
until well blended. Season with salt and pepper to taste. Set
the dressing aside.

Make the salad: Rinse and dry the greens, then tear them into
bite-size pieces. Place the greens in a large bowl, add half
of the salad dressing, and toss until the greens are coated.
Arrange the greens on a plate and top them with the tuna.
Core the tomato and cut it into eighths. Cut the string beans
in half crosswise. Place the tomato, string beans, and onion in
the bowl with the remaining salad dressing and toss to coat.
Season with salt and pepper to taste. Arrange the tomatoes,
onions, and string beans on top of the greens. If desired,
sprinkle the capers over the salad.

✳ **Fruit**

1 serving each of fruit from Group A and Group B,
see pages 67–68.

DINNER 6

✳ **Cottage Cheese and Fruit Plate**

Up to ¾ cup (up to 3 servings) nonfat or low-fat cottage cheese

Splenda or other sugar substitute (optional)

1 serving each of the fruit of your choice from Group A and
Group B (see pages 67–68)

If desired, sweeten the cottage cheese by adding sugar
substitute to taste. Spoon the cottage cheese onto a plate.
Arrange the fruit around the cottage cheese.

✳ **Side Salad**

At least 3 servings your choice of vegetables from Vegetable
Group A (see page 66)

2 servings your choice of vegetables from Vegetable Group B
(see page 67)

Salad dressing of your choice, preferably no-sugar and fat-free

Arrange the vegetables from Group A and Group B on a plate.
Top with the salad dressing.

DINNER 7

✳ **Zesty Chicken Stir-Fry**

Cooking oil spray

¼ teaspoon red pepper flakes

Low-sodium soy sauce

Up to 3 ounces (up to 3 servings) skinless, boneless chicken
or turkey breast, cut into thin strips

At least 3 servings your choice of vegetables from Vegetable
Group A (include water chestnuts and mushrooms;
see page 66)

2 servings carrots, onion, and/or snow peas (Vegetable Group B;
see page 67)

½ teaspoon minced garlic

¼ teaspoon minced peeled fresh ginger

Spray a large nonstick skillet with cooking oil spray. Add the
red pepper flakes and soy sauce to taste. Heat over medium-
high heat. Add the chicken or turkey and cook until cooked
through, about 5 minutes, stirring frequently. Add the
vegetables from Groups A and B and the garlic and ginger and
cook, stirring, until the vegetables are crisp-tender.

✳ **Fruit**

1 serving each of fruit from Group A and Group B, see pages
67–68.

6 Vegetarian Recipes

Below are six recipes that are specifically for herbivores. There
are also some vegetarian recipes, such as French Toast with
whipped YoBerry Topping (page 110), and Pancakes with Very
Berry Syrup (page 113) found within the first twenty-four meals.

VEGETARIAN BREAKFAST 1

✳ **The Shake** or **The Smoothie** (see page 50) made with
3 additional tablespoons of whey protein powder for a
total of 6 tablespoons. Or 16 ounces of low-fat milk plus
3 tablespoons of whey protein powder.

✳ **Tofu Scramble**

1½ cups (16 ounces; 4 servings) firm tofu

1 teaspoon low-sodium soy sauce

A dash each of ground turmeric, cayenne powder,
and freshly ground black pepper

2 teaspoons olive oil

3 slices tempeh bacon, chopped

2 cups broccoli florets (1 serving)

1 bell pepper, diced

½ onion, diced

2 slices of whole-grain bread, toasted

Drain the tofu, cut it into pieces, and place it in a bowl. Add the soy sauce, turmeric, cayenne, and black pepper and mash with a fork. Heat the olive oil in a small nonstick skillet, add the tempeh bacon, and cook until crisp. Add the broccoli, bell pepper, and onion and cook, stirring, until tender. Add the tofu mixture and cook, stirring, until the tofu is heated through. Serve the scramble with the whole-grain toast.

✳ Vegan cupcake or other Breakfast Sweet

(see page 69)

PROTEINS 7 SERVINGS	3 servings of low-fat or soy milk or yogurt	The Shake or The Smoothie (with 6 tablespoons of whey) or 16 ounces of milk (with 3 tablespoons of whey)
	4 servings	1½ cups of tofu and 3 slices of tempeh bacon
CARBOHYDRATES 3 SERVINGS	2 servings of bread or starches	2 slices of whole-grain toast
	1 serving	A breakfast sweet
FATS 2 SERVINGS		2 teaspoons of olive oil: Tofu Scramble

VEGETARIAN BREAKFAST 2

✳ The Shake or The Smoothie (see page 50) made with

3 additional tablespoons of whey protein powder for a
total of 6 tablespoons. Or 16 ounces of low-fat milk plus
3 tablespoons of whey protein powder.

✳ Cottage Cheese Griddle Cakes

2 tablespoons reduced-fat margarine, melted

½ cup cottage cheese (2 servings)

2 eggs (2 servings), beaten

½ cup whole-wheat flour

1 teaspoon baking powder

1 tablespoon milk

Cooking oil spray

Place the margarine and cottage cheese in a bowl and stir to mix. Stir in the eggs, followed by the whole-wheat flour, baking powder, and milk, beating until the batter is smooth and thick. Spray a griddle or nonstick skillet with cooking oil spray and heat over high heat. When very hot, using a ladle, pour scoops of the batter onto the griddle or skillet. When bubbles begin to form in the pancakes, turn them and cook until the second side is browned.

✳ Breakfast Sweet

1 serving, see page 69.

PROTEINS 7 SERVINGS	3 servings of low-fat soy milk or yogurt	The Shake or The Smoothie (with 6 tablespoons of whey) or 16 ounces of milk (with 3 tablespoons of whey)
	4 servings	½ cup of cottage cheese and 2 eggs, contained in the Cottage Cheese Griddle Cakes
CARBOHYDRATES 3 SERVINGS	2 servings of bread or starches	Contained in the Cottage Cheese Griddle Cakes
	1 serving	A breakfast sweet
FATS 2 SERVINGS		2 tablespoons reduced-fat margarine: Cottage Cheese Griddle Cakes

VEGETARIAN LUNCH 1

✳ Cheesy Spinach Salad with Strawberries

3 cups (3 servings) spinach, rinsed, dried,
and torn into bite-size pieces

1¼ cups strawberries, chopped

3 tablespoons white wine vinegar

1 tablespoon olive oil

¼ teaspoon paprika

Splenda or other sugar substitute (optional)

3 ounces (3 servings) low-fat cheese of your choice
(see page 54), torn or shredded

1 tablespoon sesame seeds

Place the spinach and strawberries in a large bowl. Place the vinegar, olive oil, and paprika in a small bowl and whisk to combine. Add sugar substitute to taste, if desired. Pour the dressing over the spinach and strawberries and toss to coat. Top the salad with the cheese and sesame seeds.

NOTE: You may substitute your favorite fat-free, low-calorie dressing for the oil and vinegar dressing here.

✳ Vegetables

At least 2 servings of vegetables from Vegetable Group B, see page 67.

VEGETARIAN LUNCH 2

✳ **The Shake** or **The Smoothie** (see page 50) made with 3 additional tablespoons of whey protein powder for a total of 6 tablespoons. Or 16 ounces of low-fat milk plus 3 tablespoons of whey protein powder.

✳ Indian Vegetable Curry

1 cup cauliflower florets

½ carrot, finely chopped

½ cup string beans, trimmed and cut in half crosswise

Cooking oil spray

⅓ large onion

¼ teaspoon cumin seeds

¼ teaspoon black mustard seeds

½ bay leaf

1⅓ jalapeño peppers, chopped
(wear plastic gloves to protect your skin when chopping)
1 clove garlic, chopped
¾ teaspoon minced peeled fresh ginger
¼ teaspoon ground cumin
¼ teaspoon curry powder

Place the cauliflower, carrot, and string beans in a microwave-safe bowl. Cover the bowl and microwave on high power until the vegetables start to soften, about 2 minutes. Drain the steamed vegetables in a colander.

Spray a large nonstick skillet with cooking oil spray and heat over medium heat. Add the onion and cook, stirring, until translucent, then stir in the cumin seeds, black mustard seeds, and the bay leaf. Cook until the seeds begin to sputter, about 30 seconds, then add the jalapeño peppers, garlic, ginger, cumin, and curry powder. Add the steamed vegetables to the skillet, reduce the heat to low, and cook until the flavors develop, about 20 minutes.

☀ **Vegetables**
At least 2 servings of vegetables from Vegetable Group A, see page 66.

☀ **Fruit**
1 serving, see pages 67–68.

VEGETARIAN DINNER 1

☀ **Bok Choy and Mushrooms**
2 cups vegetable broth
1 scallion, thinly sliced
1 clove garlic, minced
1 piece (1 inch) peeled fresh ginger, minced
12 shitake mushrooms, trimmed and sliced
8 cups chopped bok choy
¼ cup water

Pour the vegetable broth into a skillet. Add half of the scallion, garlic, and ginger. Cook, stirring, for a few minutes, then add the mushrooms and cook until tender. Place the bok choy and water in a large microwave-safe dish and microwave on high power until wilted, 2½ to 3 minutes, checking the bok choy and turning the bowl, if necessary, every minute. (You can also steam the bok choy in a steamer.) Add the mushroom mixture to the bok choy and top it with the remaining scallion, garlic, and ginger.

✳ Vegetables

At least 2 servings of vegetables from Vegetable Group B, see page 67.

✳ Fruit

1 serving each of fruit from Group A and Group B, see pages 67–68.

VEGETARIAN DINNER 2

Spicy Tofu

    1½ tablespoons soy sauce
    ¼ cup water
    1 tablespoon dry sherry
    ½ teaspoon grated peeled fresh ginger
    ¼ teaspoon crushed red pepper flakes
    Salt
    Splenda or other sugar substitute (optional)
    Up to 1½ cups (up to 12 ounces; up to 3 servings) firm tofu
    Cooking oil spray
    12 asparagus stalks, tough ends removed, stalks sliced
    2 scallions, sliced

Place the soy sauce, water, sherry, ginger, and red pepper flakes in a small bowl and whisk to mix. Season with salt and sugar substitute to taste. Set aside the soy sauce mixture. Press the excess water out of the tofu and cut it into ➡

½-inch cubes. Spray a medium-size nonstick skillet with cooking oil spray and heat over medium-high heat. When the skillet is very hot, add the tofu and cook, stirring, until golden, 3 to 4 minutes. Transfer the tofu to a bowl. Add the asparagus and scallions to the skillet and cook, stirring, until crisp-tender, 2 to 3 minutes. Transfer the asparagus and scallions to the bowl with the tofu. Add the soy sauce mixture to the skillet and cook, stirring, until bubbly, 1 to 2 minutes. Add the tofu and vegetables to the skillet and stir to coat.

❋ Vegetables

At least 2 servings of vegetables from Vegetable Group B, see page 67.

❋ Fruit

1 serving each of fruit from Group A and Group B, see pages 67–68.

STAYING
SLIM
FOR LIFE

7

AVOID
WEIGHT-LOSS
ROADBLOCKS

Congratulations! You've completed the 28-day program and are pounds and inches slimmer. You no longer crave sweets and starches, you can tuck your top into your jeans again, and your friends and coworkers can't say enough about the new, streamlined you. Enjoy those compliments and admiring (or envious) glances. You've earned them. Then float back down to earth for a dose of reality.

If you're a veteran of the diet wars, you know it's easier to lose weight than to keep it off. That's because the road of life is rarely smooth—yes, even on a diet plan that lets you eat cookies for breakfast. The unexpected pothole can drive your good intentions straight into the ditch.

For example: You're following the plan to the letter (or think you are) but your weight doesn't budge. Or you're sticking to the program all week, but slip up on the weekends. Perhaps you have a food-pushing partner or family member who continually tempts you with goodies, or maybe it's a wedding or other special event that you have to plan or attend. Vacations, stress or negative emotions, the holidays, that time of the month, dining out, simple boredom . . . Need I go on?

Each of these situations challenges your resolve. I call them roadblocks because they keep you from getting to where you want to go. But when you anticipate roadblocks, you can choose to take an entirely different route—one that keeps you on your plan.

THE SKINNY

Keeping up with a diet—between stress, holiday eating, weight-loss plateaus, and food-pushing friends or family members—can be the hardest part. You have to learn to anticipate challenges that might derail your program, and devise solutions. With a clever arsenal of tricks, you can find your way around any weight-loss "roadblock" and keep lost pounds from returning.

This chapter offers practical ways to help you strategize alternative plans—so nothing stands between you and a slimmer, healthier body. As you read, think about which roadblocks are toughest on you, then pick out one or two tips to employ the next time you encounter them. If some of these strategies help you brainstorm your own, great! That means you're *really* in the driver's seat.

ROADBLOCK #1:
"I've stopped losing weight!"

Your body is unique. Your age, gender, and, yes, genetics can impact how much you lose and how quickly, even if you eat and move the same amount as someone else. That being said, it can be disheartening to stick to your food plan and movement routine, only to see the scale stuck at the same number day after day. The good news: Weight-loss plateaus are normal and often temporary, and if you stick to your program, you will start losing again. These tips can help you bust through a plateau.

▶ **PUT AWAY THE SCALE.** If stepping on the scale and seeing no change makes you crazy, tuck it out of sight for a week. The scale often reflects the pounds of fluid you lose and gain every day rather than how much body fat you lose or gain. Also, muscle weighs more than fat, so you can lose inches of fat without losing pounds. Stay the course and you should start losing again.

▶ **STEP UP YOUR STEPS.** Add a few extra minutes to your walk. For extra motivation, clip a pedometer to your waistband each day and make a daily step goal. Pace while you chat on the phone, take the dog out for an extra walk, march in place during TV commercials. It may be enough to break the plateau.

▶ **BEWARE OF PORTION DRIFT** . . . A key cause of a weight-loss plateau is that you may be eating more than you think you are in the evenings—even with carefully measured portions. It's easy for portion sizes to creep up, and before you know it, you end up eating more than the plan prescribes. That's why it's important to understand proper portions and serving sizes.

If you've slacked off on recording your daily food intake, recommit to it. Follow the formulas—you may discover that you're taking in more than you thought.

▶ **. . . BUT DON'T SKIP MEALS!** If you restrict your calories too much for an extended period of time, your metabolism slows down to accommodate your lower caloric intake, and your body conserves fat rather than burning it for energy. Even if you work out regularly, you can hold on to body fat and end up at a plateau if you don't consume enough calories.

ROADBLOCK #2:
"I do great during the week but slip up on the weekends."

If you tend to stick to your diet during the week, but you undo all your good work come the weekend, you're not alone. Researchers at the University of North Carolina at Chapel Hill found that we consume an extra 222 calories over the course of the weekend. Here's how to stay the course on the weekends:

▶ **PLAN AROUND EVENTS, NOT FOOD.** When you break bread with friends, you eat 50 percent more food than you do by yourself, according to a Pennsylvania State University study. Shift your weekend plans to activities that don't involve eating. Ask another couple to join you at your community theater's production on Saturday night. Arrange an outing at a rollerskating rink on Sunday afternoon. If you're flying solo, visit a museum or crafts show or treat yourself to a massage.

▶ **LIMIT TV TIME.** One Lifetime or History Channel movie on a Sunday afternoon is fine. More than that and you're asking for trouble. That is, unless you're packing snacks from the approved munchies list (page 95). The longer you lounge on the couch, the more likely you are to want chips or ice cream to keep you company. Make a batch of The Stew (page 52) to sip or prep some veggies to nosh on.

▶ **HAVE A DRINK *WITH* YOUR MEAL.** It's tough to stick to any food plan when you order pre-dinner cocktails, because alcohol breaks down inhibitions. If you've kept faithfully to the Big Breakfast Diet for one month, you're allowed an occasional alcoholic beverage with your meal (I understand it's sometimes unavoidable at social gatherings). I don't recommend wine or beer, since they're packed with sugar, but one as a splurge, with dinner, is okay. Vodka- and whiskey-based drinks are preferable because they are lower in sugars. Then stick to club soda with a twist of lemon or lime.

▶ **PLAN AHEAD FOR A BIG BREAKFAST.** Between errands, kids, and chores, weekends can be too packed to accommodate a strict Big Breakfast Diet food-and-movement routine. But no matter how frantic your schedule, *don't skip breakfast.* That can trigger out-of-control cravings. Choose the Dine-and-Dash breakfast options, marked with an arrow (✈), on pages 107 through 111.

▶ **IF YOU SLIP, GET BACK ON TRACK *NOW*, NOT ON MONDAY.** If you give in to a cinnamon bun at the mall on Saturday afternoon, deal with it right away. Skip dinner. Then, eat your regular big breakfast (with a breakfast sweet) the next morning. (Whatever you do, don't ever skip breakfast to compensate—that's how you gained weight, remember?) Get back on track immediately, so you won't reactivate unhealthy eating patterns that carry over into Monday and beyond.

ROADBLOCK #3:
"I'm so bored with this diet!"

Boredom is death to a weight-loss plan. The symptoms: longing for chocolate or a gooey slice of pizza, feeling envious when you see people around you eating the foods you long for, and sneaking bites of those foods when you're alone. Even if you slip only here and there, it's enough to cause a plateau.

Although you get to eat all your favorite foods on my plan, some of my patients find it a challenge to prepare their fruits and veggies in novel ways. I present them with a challenge of my own:

to start viewing this diet as a culinary adventure. These tips can spark some inspiration—and help you stick to your food plan:

▶ **TRY A FOOD THAT MAKES YOU GO, "HUH?"** If you limit your vegetables to green beans and carrots, you're missing out on exciting flavors. Take a fresh look around the produce section—many supermarkets now offer exotic fare from faraway lands. Or visit your local Asian, Hispanic, or Middle Eastern food stores. Not quite sure what to do with starfruit, tabbouleh, or bok choy? Invest in a cookbook or two, or search culinary sites on the Web for recipes.

▶ **GET SERIOUSLY INTO SHAKES AND SMOOTHIES.** My shake and smoothie recipes (pages 50 and 52) aren't the be-all and end-all. Experiment with different combinations of fruit, milk or yogurt, flavorings, and spices. For example, you might blend milk with a shot of coffee (caf or decaf), a dash of vanilla, and a sprinkle of Splenda and cinnamon, and serve it hot or iced. You get a great-tasting beverage and your needed protein for considerably less than you'd spend at your favorite coffeehouse.

▶ **CHECK OUT AN UPSCALE SUPERMARKET.** Supermarkets such as Wegmans, Trader Joe's, and Whole Foods often have wildly exotic fruits, vegetables, and grains. Take a trip over after breakfast (when you're still full and won't over-shop) and have fun finding lunch offerings that fit in the formula.

▶ **KEEP A MENU PLANNER OF YOUR FAVORITE RECIPES.** There's no better way to keep boredom at bay than to fill a binder with recipes you absolutely love. Browse online recipe sites, print out those that appeal, and organize them by ingredient, from apples to quinoa. With your own personal cookbook full of can't-fail recipes, you're more likely to stick to the Big Breakfast Diet plan for life.

ROADBLOCK #4:

"I can't stick to a diet . . . during the holidays/on vacation/while I'm planning a special occasion/when I'm attending one . . ."

Special occasions can derail your best efforts to stick to a weight-loss plan. Planning a wedding, graduation party, or your parents' 30th anniversary disrupts your schedule, which means eating out more often, eating on the run, and missing workouts. Showers, rehearsal dinners, and work sessions can also mess up your diet.

The good news: You can eat well and enjoy special occasions; it simply takes planning. These tips can help you sail through. If you're dining out, see page 150 for dining-out tips.

DURING THE HOLIDAYS

▶ **HELP THE HOSTESS.** Invited to a holiday get-together? Lend her a helping hand. It's hard to nibble when you're busy setting the table, clearing dishes, and washing pots and pans.

▶ **ASK HER TO RECITE A RECIPE.** When she approaches you with a plate of cheese puffs or gingerbread men, say graciously, "I can't—I already stuffed myself on your delicious quiche. (You didn't, of course.) What's in that quiche, anyway?"

▶ **LOAD YOUR PLATE.** Just load it with Big Breakfast Diet fare: green salad, fruit salad, prosciutto-wrapped asparagus, shrimp, raw veggies and dip.

▶ **DESIGNATE YOURSELF THE PHOTOGRAPHER.** Wander the party and snap pictures of the merrymakers. You can't eat with a camera in your hands.

ON VACATIONS

▶ **SPLURGE ON BREAKFAST OR BRUNCH.** Most vacation destinations and cruises offer spectacular spreads. Take advantage of them during the morning hours and you won't feel "deprived" or hungry—at all.

▶ **TAKE AN ACTIVE VACATION.** Choose destinations that allow you to take walks or hikes, ride bikes, do water sports, or use the hotel tennis courts or gym.

▶ **PLAN TO *MAINTAIN* YOUR WEIGHT.** When you're on vacation, weight maintenance is a healthier and more realistic goal than weight loss.

PLANNING OR ATTENDING WEDDINGS, GRADUATIONS, ANNIVERSARIES

▶ **AS YOU PLAN, PLAN TO EAT WELL.** If you're planning your son or daughter's wedding (or your own) and meet in your home, there's no issue. Simply follow the Big Breakfast Diet parameters yourself and offer alternative fare for your guests. Keep that offering simple, and avoid making or ordering items that especially tempt you.

▶ **DINE OUT WITHOUT FILLING OUT.** If you meet in a restaurant for your planning sessions, follow the dining-out guidelines on page 150. If you'll attend one of these functions, those guidelines will help you, too.

ROADBLOCK #5:
"My friends/colleagues/ family sabotage my diet."

There's one—or more—in every family or workplace: the well-meaning (or not so well-meaning) person who pushes food on you. They shower you with tempting foods, tell you you're losing "too much weight" or that you "look sick," or predict that you will just regain all the weight you've lost. Sometimes, they complain that you spend "too much time" working out.

This is a difficult situation, but there are ways to get around it. The key: standing your ground in a pleasant way rather than a confrontational one.

AT FAMILY GATHERINGS

▶ **JUST SAY NO.** When a food pusher offers you a food that's not on your plan, simply smile and give a pleasant "No, thanks"—no explanation or excuses necessary. If they persist, repeat "No, thanks." Do not accept the plate, and hand it back with a smile.

▶ **BRING A HEALTHY DISH.** When you're invited to your mother's for Sunday dinner, bring a huge bowl of green salad or fruit salad to share. Take a few spoonfuls of the other offerings and move them around on your plate, so you get to "eat" with the family. When she pushes leftovers on you, accept them graciously— maybe they can be incorporated into tomorrow's big breakfast!

AT WORK

▶ **DO THE CAKE FAKEOUT.** Cake often seems mandatory at office birthday parties or celebrations. It's not. Just pass the plate to another colleague, or politely decline. If you think your refusal will draw attention and perhaps resentment, accept a small piece (if you know you can resist eating it right away). Then wrap it up and save it for the morning. If it still says "Eat me!" in the A.M., make it your breakfast sweet.

AT HOME

▶ **HAVE A HEART-TO-HEART WITH YOUR SPOUSE.** Your partner may fear that if you lose weight, you'll get more attention from others. First, reassure your partner that you love him or her and ask for support. Next, gently suggest that the food he or she brings home doesn't help your health, and that it may affect your children's future health as well.

▶ **KEEP JUNK FOOD OUT.** Ask your partner to eat junk food away from home, rather than bringing it into the house. If junk food continues to appear, carry the treats into the garage or garden shed every time you find them. It'll get the message across. And stay strong. You're doing something good for yourself.

ROADBLOCK #6:
"I'm following the plan exactly, but I'm gaining again!"

Portion drift might be the problem here. If you eat just 100 extra calories per day, you'll gain 10 pounds in one year! These tips can help you check to see if you're eating more than you think. It helps to know your terms. A *portion* size is the amount offered in packaged foods *or* the amount you choose to put on your plate. A *serving* is a standard unit of food, such as one cup or one ounce. To control your *portions*, you've got to be aware of *serving size*.

GET A GRIP ON SERVING SIZE

▶ **READ LABELS.** The nutrition-facts label that's on almost all packaged foods tells you what one serving size is and how many calories that serving contains.

▶ **MEASURE, MEASURE, MEASURE.** Before you eat, break out the measuring cups and spoons. Use them to place one serving-size amount of food (including salad dressing) on your plate.

This way you get to see what one serving of that food looks like, compared to how much you typically eat.

► **USE YOUR PALM AS A GUIDE** . . . If you don't have a scale or measuring cup available, use the "palm method." From chicken breasts to cooked veggies or fresh fruit, just about every correct portion size fits in your cupped palm.

► **OR USE VISUALS.** One serving of protein (1 ounce) is about the size of a small box of matches; one serving of cheese (1 ounce), the size of a die; one serving of cooked veggies or fresh fruit, the size of a baseball.

► **PLAY THE RAINBOW GAME.** Hate measuring? See how many colors you can fit on your plate. Leafy greens and broccoli, red tomatoes, orange carrots or bell pepper, yellow squash, just a sprinkle of white feta or goat cheese . . . Use the same trick with fruit. Focus on creating a colorful plate of fruits and veggies, and forget about measuring, except for dressing.

MANAGE PORTION SIZE

► **DON'T EAT FROM THE BOX OR BAG.** I recommend that you don't take meals or snacks in front of the TV, period—it leads to mindless eating. But if you do, put the amount you plan to eat onto a plate or into a bowl or container. Don't eat straight from the package.

► **USE SMALLER PLATES.** The smaller your plate, the smaller your portions.

► **PAY MORE FOR SINGLE-SERVING BAGS.** That way you know when you've had one serving.

► **BE ESPECIALLY CONSCIOUS OF YOUR BREAKFAST SWEET.** Enjoy anything you like—cookies, cake, pie, chocolate—but be vigilant about portion size.

ROADBLOCK #7:

"I'm so angry/lonely/sad... a cookie will help."

In a perfect world, you'd eat only when you were physically hungry. Alas, many people who struggle with their weight have learned to soothe any uncomfortable emotions, including anxiety, anger, or sadness, with food—and they pay a high physical and emotional price.

When you're an emotional eater, it's hard to stick to a diet because you have learned to use food to manage your feelings. While addressing the root causes of emotional eating is beyond the scope of this book, there are many wonderful books you can find at your local library or bookstore that address the topic. You might also consider working with a counselor who specializes in compulsive overeating as you follow my plan. In the meantime, these tools may help, at least in the short run.

► **MUNCH.** There is a list of approved munchies on page 95 that are essentially "free foods." If you need your jaw to be working, but can't afford for it to go to your waist, chow down, guilt-free, on some freebies. You'll satisfy your need to eat without derailing your diet.

► **CONNECT WITH OTHERS.** Create a support system. If you're on the diet with a friend, check in with him or her when you feel a craving coming on. A simple phone call may help break the tendency to comfort yourself with food.

► **BURN OFF A BINGE.** Fighting off the urge to raid the cookie jar? Get moving. Roughhouse with your dog, clean a closet, rake a huge pile of leaves, fold the laundry, or take a short walk. Just get your body moving.

9 Ways to Outwit the Dining-Out Trap

Going out to dinner and sticking to the Big Breakfast Diet principles doesn't have to be a hassle. Follow these tactics and you'll do just fine.

1. **REVIEW THE MENU FROM HOME.** If you're dining at a chain restaurant, check its website; most post the nutritional information for their menus. Decide on your meal before you leave home—or, conversely, how you will ask the server to prepare your entrée for you.

2. **START WITH AN APPETIZER.** To me, the perfect start to a perfect meal is a shrimp cocktail. Hold the cocktail sauce and squeeze on a bit of fresh lemon, or take a tablespoon or so of sauce as a splurge. Or opt to have your dessert first: a plump bowl of fresh fruit salad.

3. **IGNORE THE BREAD BASKET.** Unless you're at a restaurant that serves crusty artisanal bread, most bread isn't worth the carbs. But if the restaurant is known for its bread, and it's truly

---

THAT TIME OF THE MONTH

If PMS tends to derail your diet—and your weight loss—you're not alone. A recent study that analyzed dietary associations with PMS found that women with PMS were 245 percent more likely to have an increased level of refined sugar intake, 79 percent consumed more salt, and 77 percent had lower levels of magnesium, a mineral that helps break down estrogen and metabolize carbohydrates.

The Big Breakfast Diet plan may help reduce cravings associated with PMS because it's high in hunger-satisfying protein. Also, let's not forget that you get to indulge your sweet tooth (and fat tooth, and carb tooth) at breakfast! But if cravings do hit, try these tips:

exceptional, travel with a ziplock bag so you can take a slice to go. Seal it up so it stays fresh and moist until breakfast.

4. SPEAK UP FOR SUBSTITUTIONS. If your entrée comes with fries or cole slaw, request a salad, dressing on the side, or grilled or roasted veggies instead—pay extra if you have to. Or if you get three side orders with your entrée, ask your waiter for a triple order of steamed, grilled, or roasted veggies.

5. PRACTICE PREVENTIVE PORTION CONTROL. Because most restaurants offer gigantic portions, ask your server to box half your entrée (except for the veggies) and serve the other half.

6. USE THE DIP-AND-SPEAR METHOD FOR SALADS. When you order your grilled-chicken salad or spinach salad, ask for dressing on the side. Dip your fork into the dressing, then spear a forkful of greens. You'll be surprised at how little dressing you actually need to enjoy its flavor.

7. TREAT YOURSELF TO SEAFOOD. I find that few of my patients cook seafood at home, so it's a treat when you dine out,

---

- ▶ A few days before your period, limit your salt intake to reduce bloating and water weight gain.

- ▶ Get plenty of sleep—about eight hours a night. (You should be doing that anyway!)

- ▶ If PMS stress hits, take a walk around the block instead of to the vending machine for a chocolate bar.

- ▶ If a craving hits in the afternoon or at night, wait 15 to 30 minutes to see if it passes. If it doesn't, see how long you can wait it out.

Your monthly cycle is not something you can avoid, so the best remedy is to be prepared. Drink plenty of water, stay active, and keep stress to a minimum.

MENU READING 101

Restaurant food can absolutely fit in the Big Breakfast Diet formulas. Knowing what *words* you should avoid will help guide you away from *foods* you should avoid. Here are some common menu descriptions that suggest lower and higher fat content.

LOWER FAT CONTENT

grilled • poached • broiled • braised • baked • roasted • boiled • steamed • au jus • stir-fried • dry (broiled in wine)

HIGHER FAT CONTENT

fried • buttered • breaded • au gratin • crispy • rich • creamed, creamy • Béarnaise or Hollandaise sauce • Parmesan

especially the more exotic varieties such as Chilean sea bass or lobster. Request that your fish or shellfish be baked, broiled, sautéed, poached, steamed, or grilled, and that it be prepared without extra oil or butter. Nix sauces, or request them on the side.

8. TEMPT YOURSELF WITH LEAN MEAT OR POULTRY. Your best bets include skinless chicken breasts, pork loin, and beef sirloin. Again, request that it be baked, broiled, grilled, poached, or roasted without extra butter or oil.

9. HAVE DESSERT RAW. For a sweet ending to your meal, order a dish of fresh-fruit compote—any fruits from Fruit Group A contain only 5 to 10 percent sugar. If you stick to the recommended serving sizes, you can have these moderate sweets in the evening (sweetened with Splenda, if you like).

8

THE NO-SWEAT EXERCISE CURE

've treated hundreds of overweight men and women over the years. What I've learned is that if you want to see a dieter fail in his or her attempt to lose weight, just tell the person to exercise.

Physical activity is a key part of a successful weight-loss plan. It also benefits your cardiovascular health and helps reduce your risk of diabetes, osteoporosis, and other diseases. Furthermore, studies show that people who get physically active *and* watch their diet are the most successful "losers."

But let's face it: People who struggle with their weight often avoid exercise. In fact, many of my own patients feared that I'd tell them they had to huff and puff at the gym for an hour a day. They couldn't have exercised that long even if they wanted to, and most of them didn't want to. And they certainly didn't want to be on a cardio machine next to someone with a perfect body.

The good news is, you don't have to sweat buckets on a treadmill or elliptical trainer to lose weight. Really, you don't.

THE SKINNY

To lose weight and keep it off, you've got to move your body. In just 10 to 20 minutes a day, you can burn calories, build muscle, and improve your body's sensitivity to insulin. So get ready, get set, and choose one of two options—a daily walk or one or two 10-minute sessions of activity.

Here's a fact that may surprise you: Physical activity accounts for just 12 percent—at best—of the typical person's daily caloric expenditure. The remaining 88 percent is used to sustain life—digest food, breathe, keep the heart beating. What this means is that people who consume 1,500 calories a day will burn maybe 180 of them through exercise, unless they're world-class athletes.

That's why I won't make you "exercise" on my fitness plan. All I want you to do—all you *need* to do—is to start by moving your body for 20 minutes a day. The Big Breakfast Diet food plan will take care of the rest.

If you're already involved in a fitness routine you enjoy, stick with it. If not, get ready to view "exercise" in a whole new way. You can choose between two fun, easy 20-minute plans, and I use the term "plan" loosely. You can even break those 20 minutes into two 10-minute blocks, if you like.

Short and sweet, fun and flexible—"exercise" doesn't get much easier than this. After you lose weight and gain energy, you can become even more active if you like. But that's the beauty of my plan—a little movement will net you big rewards.

Three Good Reasons to Get a Move On

If you're like most people, you know all too well that, at the start of a diet, you lose weight quickly. But inevitably, the weight loss slows down, even if you stick to your diet religiously. If you cheat even a little, you regain those lost pounds almost immediately. It's frustrating, but the important thing is to ask is: Why?

It's simple. As you lose weight, your metabolism slows. Think of those extra 15, 20, or more pounds as a heavy suitcase. As strange as it seems, you use a good amount of energy (calories) to drag that "luggage" around. When you lose weight, it's like you've exchanged that heavy suitcase for a lighter carry-on bag. And a smaller bag doesn't take as much energy to carry.

If you follow the old "diet-hard-but-don't-move" plan, you will lose weight at first. But as time goes on, you'll also lose muscle, which will make it harder to *continue* to lose weight. In fact, diet without exercise can slow metabolism by up to 30 percent. So to keep your weight loss on track, move it! Here's what you stand to gain (and it's not pounds).

THE MANY BENEFITS OF
MOVEMENT

Don't move your body just to lose weight. Do it to improve your physical, mental, and emotional well-being, as well. To get yourself motivated, ponder the known rewards of regular physical activity:

- ▶ Reduces feelings of depression and anxiety
- ▶ Improves self-esteem and feelings of well-being
- ▶ Helps protect bones, muscles, and joints
- ▶ Builds muscular strength and endurance
- ▶ Enhances flexibility
- ▶ Improves posture
- ▶ Protects against cardiovascular disease, type 2 diabetes, and some types of cancer
- ▶ Helps control blood pressure

YOU'LL BURN CALORIES. It takes energy (calories) to move your body, whether the movement is generated in the gym or in your yard as you rake leaves. If you're physically active, not only will you burn more calories, you'll raise your basal metabolic rate (BMR) for up to 48 hours after the activity. In other words, up to two days after your brisk walk or raking session, you burn more calories than usual even when you're lounging on the couch watching TV. This elevation in BMR speeds up the fat loss promoted by the Big Breakfast Diet plan.

YOU'LL IMPROVE YOUR BODY'S SENSITIVITY TO INSULIN. As I mentioned earlier, overweight people have a chemical blockage in their muscle cells that affects the action of insulin. As a result, energy (glucose) from food doesn't go to the muscles where it's needed. It goes to the belly, backside, hips, and thighs as body fat. Physical activity reduces that blockage in muscle cells, which makes them more sensitive to insulin's action.

YOU'LL INCREASE YOUR MUSCLE MASS. The more muscle tissue you have, the higher your BMR. On the other hand, when you're inactive, you lose muscle tissue, which drastically slows your metabolism (because pound for pound, muscle burns more calories than fat does). If you follow my recommendations, you'll build a bit of muscle, which will help keep your BMR humming along.

Turn Exercise into Playtime

Chances are, when you were a kid you loved to exercise. Of course, you didn't *call* it exercise. You played tag or rode your bike. But at some point we began to equate moving our bodies with drudgery rather than pleasure.

It's time to make being active fun again, or at least bearable. A good way to begin: Discard the idea that exercise has to be a chore to do you good.

Cardiovascular exercise ("cardio" for short) isn't defined by how sweaty and exhausted you are when you're done. It simply makes you breathe a *little* harder and makes your heart beat a little faster. Sure, an hour on the treadmill can do that, but wouldn't you rather play Frisbee with your dog in the yard, dig in your garden, or enjoy a day at the roller rink or a night of square-dancing?

"Intensity" is how hard your body works during cardiovascular exercise. Research shows that moderate-intensity exercise, for example a daily brisk walk or bicycle ride, offers the same health benefits as a high-intensity exercise like jogging. When you exercise at a moderate intensity, you're working hard enough to raise your heart rate and break a light sweat, yet still have the breath to carry on a conversation.

According to the Centers for Disease Control and Prevention, most people need to exercise an hour a day, most days of the week, to manage body weight and maintain weight loss. That's a noble goal, but in my clinical experience, most people don't have the time or inclination to do this. So all I want you to do is move for 20 minutes a day. You can walk, dance, weed your garden, sled down a hill with your kids. Do whatever you wish, just *do*.

This small amount of movement doesn't just burn calories and get glucose into your muscles, it also protects your cardiovascular health. Research conducted at Brigham and Women's Hospital in Boston found that women who exercised just two hours a week— that's 17 minutes a day!—reduced their risk of heart disease and stroke by 27 percent. Other research links physical activity with a lower risk of osteoporosis, diabetes, and some cancers.

So move your body just a little, and you'll reap huge rewards. You'll also have fun, because there are so many ways to get moving that will bring you pleasure.

Your (Easy) Activity Options

To best improve insulin sensitivity and glucose control, you want to choose movement that works your buttocks and thighs. That means you can walk, ride your bicycle, dance, do martial arts . . . the list is long. As these large muscles work, they tap into the glucose in your blood for energy. Since this glucose won't linger in your bloodstream anymore, it won't be stored as body fat.

OPTION #1: THE 20-MINUTE WALK

Walking is safe, gentle, easy on your joints, and doesn't require fancy equipment. You can do it alone, with a friend, or with a group. A brisk walk can also reduce stress and boost your mood and your energy levels.

Research has shown that a person needs to burn around 2,000 to 3,000 calories from physical activity every week to control body weight. That works out to 60 to 90 minutes per day—an unrealistic goal, I've found, for most people who struggle with extra pounds.

I'm asking you to walk just 20 minutes because, in my experience, that's a realistic amount of time, at least in the initial stages of a weight-loss program. If you are not currently fit enough to walk 20 minutes, start with 10 and add to your time each week.

As you walk, don't concern yourself with how many calories you're burning. The answer is usually "less than you think." The important thing is that you're getting blood glucose into your muscles where it's needed. Walk as briskly as you comfortably can. (If you're huffing and puffing, slow down.)

MY PRESCRIPTION: Take a 20-minute walk after lunch or dinner, or sneak out of the office after 3 P.M. to beat the moodiness and fatigue of the dreaded midafternoon slump. Or take two brisk 10-minute walks per day.

If you *want* to walk 30 minutes or even more, you may—but only if you want to. It's easy to get in those extra minutes, too. For example, you might do two 15-minute walks a day, and throw in mini-walks as time and opportunity permit. Does your child walk to his bus stop? Walk with him or her. At the mall, take the stairs instead of the elevator, or when you go to the supermarket, pick the parking spot farthest away from the entrance—let the other shoppers fight for the nearest ones.

OPTION #2: THE 10-MINUTE MOVES

Can't walk or don't want to? Have an especially busy day ahead? This option is for you, especially if you like the idea of breaking up your activity into manageable 10-minute blocks.

If you think a 10-minute burst of activity can't possibly help you lose weight, think again. Research has shown that sprinkling your day with 10-minute bouts of moderate-intensity physical activity can be just as effective as a half-hour workout.

MY PRESCRIPTION: Do any one of the activities below for 10 minutes once or twice a day. If you're enjoying yourself, feel free to do one 20-minute session (or more, to your comfort level). For more ideas on how to fit 10-minute bursts of activity into your day, see the box on page 160.

10-MINUTE MOVE 1: EXERCISE YOUR GREEN THUMB. Experts have dubbed gardening "green exercise" for good reason. When you dig and weed, and mulch and hoe, you're engaging in moderate-intensity physical activity. As a bonus, you can grow some of the fruits and veggies you enjoy on my plan.

10-MINUTE MOVE 2: SHAKE YOUR BOOTY. Turn on the stereo and dance like crazy right there in the living room. Or go out for a night of country line dancing, or join a tango or swing-dancing class. You don't have to do a strenuous form of dance like hip-hop, either. You can waltz, hula, even belly dance if you like.

10-MINUTE MOVE 3: MOVE IT WITH Wii FIT. If you tend to get bored with the same-old same-old fitness routine, consider this option.

EXERCISE
YOU DON'T EVEN NOTICE
AT HOME:

▶ Join a neighborhood walking group—you'll enjoy the camaraderie and get your walk in!

▶ Play with your kids—push your baby in the stroller, play tag or jump in the leaves in the backyard, build a snowman, go on a bike ride.

▶ Walk the soccer or softball field sidelines as you cheer your kids on.

▶ Take your dog for a quick walk around the block.

▶ Wash your car by hand instead of at the drive-through car wash.

▶ Mow the lawn with your old push mower.

AT WORK:

▶ Replace your usual coffee break with a brisk 10-minute walk.

▶ Get off the bus or subway one stop early and walk the rest of the way.

▶ Take part in an exercise program at work or a nearby gym.

▶ Join the office softball or bowling team.

You can do yoga, walk a tightrope, downhill ski, box, dance, hula hoop, and more. And since you can "play" with more than one person, you can get your kids involved in the fun.

10-MINUTE MOVE 4: TRY TAI CHI. This centuries-old Chinese practice exercises the mind and body in a series of gentle, flowing postures. Because it's low impact, it's a good choice for people who carry extra pounds.

Tai chi also speaks to the mental aspect of overweight. When you practice tai chi, you connect with your body, which can help improve your body image, reduce stress, and give you the calm and insight you need to make healthy food choices.

Your All-Day Metabolism-Revving Prescription

On my plan you eat to suit your body's natural rhythms in order to accelerate your metabolism and burn body fat. Ideally, you'll be physically active in accordance with these rhythms as well.

I strongly recommend that you get in your 20 minutes of movement in the afternoon or early evening, at least three hours before bed. (I'll explain why in a moment.) But let's discuss morning workouts first.

Many people work out early in the morning either because it suits their schedule or because they find that if they don't do it first thing, it won't get done.

It's not the ideal time to exercise because cardiovascular rhythms and adrenaline are at their highest, but if that's when you have time it's fine—but you should keep your exercise low-impact and you *must* eat first. Not much—a few servings of solid protein will do. (You can enjoy your Shake or Smoothie post-workout.) Your muscles need it to guard against those protein-gobbling morning hormones, adrenaline and cortisol.

As you recall, cortisol helps your body obtain blood glucose from proteins. If you don't eat within 15 minutes of waking up, that alarm system in your brain activates, directing the body to get the protein it needs from your muscle tissue. Add a walk on top of your morning fast and you break down even more muscle tissue. In fact, studies of marathon runners have shown that when they fast before they run, they lose twice the amount of muscle proteins during the first hour than during the rest of their run!

Eat some of your protein servings first thing in the morning— a quick egg-white scramble, a few servings of cheese, 4 ounces of your morning shake or smoothie—and your muscle tissue will be spared. But to keep your metabolic furnace blazing brightly, do your 20-minute walk or workout in the late afternoon or early evening, if you can. With sunset, cortisol and adrenaline fall, while hormones that utilize fat reserves rise. Walk or work out in the late afternoon or early evening and you help your body utilize fat reserves for fuel and protect muscle mass.

DIFFERENT WEIGHT, DIFFERENT BURN

Every little bit of activity affects your health—some activities are simply more efficient ways to burn calories. The chart at right shows the approximate caloric expenditure in 30 minutes of physical activity. Because the heavier you are, the more calories you burn, three different weights are provided: 125, 155, and 185 pounds. If you weigh more or less than this, you'll burn more or fewer calories.

ACTIVITY	CALORIES BURNED		
AT HOME	**125 LB**	**155 LB**	**185 LB**
Sleeping	19	23	28
Watching TV	23	28	33
Sitting: reading	34	42	50
Standing	38	47	56
Cooking	75	93	111
Childcare: bathing, feeding, etc.	105	130	155
Heavy cleaning: washing car, windows	135	167	200

IN THE YARD OR GARDEN

Gardening, *general*	135	167	200
Planting seedlings or shrubs	120	149	178
Planting trees	135	167	200
Raking lawn	120	149	178
Bagging grass or leaves	120	149	178
Mowing lawn *(push or power)*	135	167	200
Shoveling snow by hand	180	223	266
Operating snow blower *(walking)*	135	167	200
Carrying or stacking wood	150	186	222
Chopping or splitting wood	180	223	266

AT PLAY

Badminton	135	167	200
Dancing *(disco, ballroom, square)*	165	205	244
Dancing *(fast, ballet)*	180	223	266
Golf, *carrying clubs*	165	205	244
Golf, *using cart*	105	130	155

ACTIVITY	CALORIES BURNED		
	125 LB	155 LB	185 LB
Hiking	180	223	266
Horseback riding	120	149	178
Ice-skating	210	260	311
Martial arts *(judo, karate, etc.)*	300	372	444
Rollerblading	210	260	311
Skiing, *cross-country*	240	298	355
Skiing, *downhill*	180	223	266
Snorkeling	150	186	222
Snowshoeing	240	298	355
Swimming, general	180	223	266
Swimming, laps	300	372	444
Tai chi	120	149	178
Tennis	210	260	311
White-water rafting or kayaking	150	186	222

WALKING, RUNNING, AND CYCLING

	125 LB	155 LB	185 LB
Walking, 3.5 mph *(17 min/mi)*	120	149	178
Walking, 4 mph *(15 min/mi)*	135	167	200
Walking, 4.5 mph *(13 min/mi)*	150	186	222
Running, 5 mph *(12 min/mi)*	240	298	355
Running, 6 mph *(10 min/mi)*	300	372	444
Running, 6.7 mph *(9 min/mi)*	330	409	488
Mountain biking	255	316	377
Bicycling, 12–13.9 mph	240	298	355
Bicycling, 14–15.9 mph	300	372	444
Bicycling, 16–19 mph	360	446	533

9

STAY SLIM FOR LIFE: MAINTAINING YOUR WEIGHT LOSS

Now that you've followed the Big Breakfast Diet plan for a month, you should notice a few striking changes. You're no longer controlled by Fat Brain, a protein-packed breakfast has become a habit, and dinner has become a mere formality. You sail through your day with more energy, a brighter mood, and virtually no hunger or afternoon and nighttime cravings. Best of all, you can zip up your favorite pair of jeans again.

So how do you maintain your goal weight for life? You continually work on your ability to think slim.

The principles of weight maintenance are much like those of weight loss: Eat in sync and move your body each day. And like weight loss, weight maintenance requires a long-term commitment.

If you've always thought of dieting as a means to an end, rather than as a permanent lifestyle change, rethink that notion. You can't let all the good habits you've picked up during this

THE SKINNY

The formula for successful weight maintenance isn't much different from the formula for successful weight loss: Eat in sync and move your body each day. However, diets are like a sprint: You focus on swift or immediate results. Maintenance is like a marathon: You've got to settle in for the long haul and forget about the finish line, because there is none. If you can adopt the 5 Principles of Weight Maintenance, you'll keep your newly slim body for life.

month on the diet fall by the wayside now that you've reached your goal. If you do, those extra pounds will return. Day by day, week by week, you must consistently eat well, and abandon the eating habits that got you fat in the first place. That means you must make eating in sync as much a daily habit as brushing your teeth.

On the Big Breakfast Diet plan, you have two options to maintain your weight.

OPTION 1: Continue to enjoy your large breakfast in order to keep your metabolism humming and control hunger and addiction. To your lunch, add one portion of starches (⅔ cup brown rice or other whole grain, a medium baked potato, or a slice of whole-grain bread). Keep dinner the same as on the diet, but you can be more flexible in consuming your three servings (and even add one more serving) of lean protein. While in optimum weight loss mode, you shouldn't have even felt hungry for dinner, but in maintenance mode, you're cleared to eat the protein servings if you really feel the need.

OPTION 2: Most of my patients prefer this option. Continue the basic Big Breakfast Diet plan six days a week. On Day 7, have a free day. Eat what you want, at any time of the day. Dine at your favorite restaurant, for example, and enjoy a glass of wine and dessert. Your weight will be up a few pounds the next day, but when you return to the diet in the following days you will drop those pounds easily.

5 Principles of Weight Maintenance

#1 STEP ON THE SCALE EVERY DAY

Many weight-loss experts advise against daily weigh-ins—scale hopping can frustrate you, they contend. I agree that when you're trying to lose, it makes sense to weigh in once a week. Once you hit your goal weight, though, things change. You've worked so hard to get to your goal weight. Now you must defend it, and in this case the scale is your ally.

So once you hit your goal weight, step on the scale every morning, after you use the bathroom and before your breakfast. Also, draw a line in the sand: Don't ever go more than two pounds above your goal weight. Ever, ever. Go back on the basic plan until you lose them. It's easier to lose two pounds than five or ten.

If you step on the scale the morning after a free day, you'll probably weigh more. Don't panic. You'll lose the extra weight in the next few days, because you'll be back on the basic plan. But if those pounds hang around for a week or more, make sure you're following your maintenance plan—and the recommendations below—to the letter.

#2 DON'T SLACK OFF AT BREAKFAST TIME

Many experts stress the importance of portion control; lack of it is what packs the weight on. That's true—if you're not eating in sync. If you are, portion sizes take care of themselves.

Remember, on this plan, there's no need to count calories. Your focus during both weight loss and maintenance is to eat breakfast exactly as I prescribe.

If you eat enough protein and a couple of carb servings at breakfast, and get in that craving-crushing breakfast sweet, you simply won't experience hunger or cravings. If you do, chances are good that you didn't eat a true Big Breakfast Diet breakfast.

It sounds counterintuitive, but always make sure that you consume *at least seven* servings of protein at your morning meal. And never, ever give up your breakfast sweet to save calories. You need the protein to cut hunger and speed metabolism, and the sweet to keep your serotonin at above-cravings levels.

#3 CONTINUE THOSE BRISK WALKS

You began your walking program 28 days ago—enough time, research shows, to have made lacing up your sneakers a habit. That's good, because walking doesn't just help you lose weight. It helps you keep it off, too.

Fully 76 percent of people tracked through the National Weight Control Registry—folks who have lost an average of 66 pounds and kept it off for five-plus years—walk regularly for exercise. If walking works for those "losers," it will work for you. So tie up your sneakers and get moving!

To reinforce your walking habit, make this activity about your quality of life rather than about your weight. When you walk to destress and add much needed "me time" to your frantic schedule, this 30 minutes becomes an oasis in your day rather than just another chore tacked on to your to-do list. Refresh your motivation often. Treat yourself to fun-to-use gadgets, such as walking poles or a pedometer. Seek out new walking paths. If you can, walk rather than drive to a favorite destination, such as a cozy local bookstore. Have fun with your walking program. When your motivation is to keep your walk fresh and ever-challenging, you're more likely to stick with it.

BIG-TIME LOSERS—
FOLLOW THEIR LEAD

Almost 20 years ago, the University of Colorado's National Weight Control Registry began tracking more than 3,000 regular people who lost more than 60 pounds and kept it off for more than five years.

Professor James O. Hill and his team have zeroed in on four things these successful "losers" tend to do. Among them:

▶ Weigh in every day.
▶ Eat breakfast every day.
▶ Keep a food journal.
▶ Be physically active for about an hour a day (walking counts).

If this sounds challenging, here's some encouragement: Only one third of the participants described maintaining their weight loss as hard. One third described it as moderately easy, while the remaining third said it was a breeze. In fact, 42 percent reported that maintenance was easier than initially losing the weight!

#4 SLEEP ENOUGH, SLEEP WELL

As you learned earlier, how much sleep you get, and how well you sleep, can affect your weight. Unfortunately, sleep is one of the first things we give up when life gets complicated. Without at least eight hours of sound, good-quality sleep, your ability to concentrate and make healthy choices is also compromised.

Sleep-deprived people have an increased risk of health problems, including obesity. They eat more because they're hungrier; they're awake longer and may be tempted by foods everywhere they go. They often consume far more calories than they burn in the extra hours they're awake. What's more, when you don't get enough restorative deep or slow-wave sleep, your levels of HGH, which helps your body burn stored fat, may dip.

Of course, snoozing a few hours longer each night won't keep you slim on its own—you'll still need to eat in sync and keep active. But each time you're tempted to stay up past your bedtime, remember that 65 percent of Americans are overweight and 63 percent of people don't get eight hours of sleep a night. That's a great reason to crawl into bed at the end of a long, hard day: When your body doesn't hunger for sleep, it won't hunger for cookies or chips, either.

#5 STAY SERIOUS ABOUT STRESS CONTROL

There are times in life where weight maintenance is more difficult. You quit smoking or change jobs. You face relationship or financial difficulties. When you're stressed out, every task becomes more challenging. You may chain yourself to your desk to make your deadline rather than get out for your walk. Worse, you may start to skip breakfast or seek comfort in food, which will put you on the fast track to extra pounds. Regaining the weight you struggled to lose will only add to your stress.

It's vital to stick to the healthy habits you know will control your weight—even when you don't want to. Easier said than done, but when you take time out for relaxation and exercise, you're less likely to fall back to the habits that led to your initial weight gain.

No matter how squeezed your schedule or how much stress you may feel, turn to activities that comfort you rather than to food. Get enough sleep. Each and every day, do one thing that gives you pleasure, no matter how small. Strive to retain your ability to seek out and experience pleasure, and make yourself and your health your first priority.

NO PAIN, NO REGAIN:
Common Maintenance
Challenges Solved

Sticking to a weight-loss plan comes with its own set of challenges. So does maintenance. Here are a trio of issues you might face while on maintenance, along with suggested solutions.

▶ **PROBLEM:** There's no time for breakfast, so you grab whatever's at hand without following the Big Breakfast Diet formula.

SOLUTION: Keep a few cans of a high-protein shake in your refrigerator for rushed mornings. Sip while you dress and apply makeup. Before you head out the door, slap together a sandwich: sliced ham or turkey and cheese with mayo, lettuce, and tomato. Munch on your way to work (if you commute), or wrap it up to eat when you get to the office.

▶ **PROBLEM:** You skipped breakfast and lunch, and now, at 3 P.M., you crave a high-carb coffee drink from the specialty coffee shop in your building, or a doughnut from the office vending machine.

SOLUTION: Dig into your desk drawer for the protein bars or single-serving packages of unsalted almonds you've been saving for such emergencies. Then eat your regular dinner.

▶ **PROBLEM:** You absolutely, positively cannot bear the thought of another sandwich.

SOLUTION: Expand your definition of a sandwich. It doesn't have to be cold. It doesn't even have to be made with sandwich bread. Think grilled bread, roasted veggies, exotic ingredients. The only must: two servings of carbs, seven of protein. Try the super easy, spicy fish-taco "sandwich" on page 108 that fits the bill.

APPENDIX 1

THE FORMULAS

Each formula, used in conjunction with the Servings List (pages 54 through 70) is your guide to the Big Breakfast Diet. Use this at-a-glance cheat sheet to follow the formulas as you build your own meals.

BREAKFAST FORMULA (PAGE 75)

7 servings protein
  (2 of which must be milk- or yogurt-based)
2 servings carbohydrate
2 servings fat
1 serving breakfast sweet

LUNCH FORMULA (PAGE 92)

3 servings protein
  (none of which may be milk- or yogurt-based)
3 servings from Vegetable Group A
2 servings from Vegetable Group B
1 serving from Fruit Groups A, B, C, or D

DINNER FORMULA (PAGE 94)

0–3 servings protein
Unlimited servings from Vegetable Group A
2 servings from Vegetable Group B
1 serving from Fruit Group A
1 serving from Fruit Group B

THE FIRST 28 DAYS

I t's time for action! Use the following pages to design your meals and workouts and to reflect on behaviors that help or hinder your success—so you can brainstorm possible solutions to any challenges that arise. You can also track your progress: inches lost, confidence gained, and goals met.

Start on Day 1. Write as much or as little as you wish, but do write every day. At the end of each week, look for patterns. Note what time you ate each meal and how hungry you were when you were eating it. Did you run into any challenges when planning or eating breakfast? How was your energy level the rest of the day? Do you tend to follow the program faithfully all week, only to fall off the wagon on Friday or Saturday? Brainstorm ways to make weekends easier. Do cravings seem to crop up whenever you're stressed or tired? Review the Cures for Cravings, and pick several new ones to try the next time you're overwhelmed or exhausted.

You don't have to write a novel to benefit from this workbook. Even writing a line or two each day can help you gain new insights into how you *really* feel about food, your weight, and your body, which will make it that much easier for you to stick to the program. Remember—knowledge is power!

BIG BREAKFAST DIET
SAMPLE DAY

DATE: *January 1*

MY WEIGHT
TODAY: *180 lb.*

MY WAIST
TODAY: *44"*

MENU

Write down your meal plan for each day. Then take notes on meals
you'd like to repeat and meals you'd like to adjust. For example, if
you find you're hungry before lunchtime, make a note to increase
your proteins at breakfast on subsequent days. If you really love a
recipe you tried for dinner, make a note to have it again soon!

MENU NOTES

BREAKFAST *fruit smoothie*

country style scramble

2 slices toast w/ butter   * still hungry at 10:30;
try peanut butter
instead!

chocolate doughnut

LUNCH *chef salad, kiwi*

½ cup OJ   * ate cup of
The Stew as
afternoon snack

DINNER *lemon-lime scallops*   * yum!

NOTES I'm not used to eating sweets for breakfast so
I almost forgot to eat one this morning. Later, out of
instinct, I bought M&M's from the snack machine but
convinced myself I could save them for breakfast tomorrow!

> Go confidently in the direction of
> your dreams! Live the life you've
> imagined.
>
> —*Thoreau*

WORKOUT

Did you get in your physical activity? In this section, reflect on
your daily walk or 10-minute workout(s). Be sure to record what
time you took your exercise, your mood at the time, and whether
you noticed improvements in strength or energy. Suggested
topics: How did you feel during exercise—tired or energized,
motivated or blah? If you tried a new activity, did you enjoy it?
If you skipped your walk or workout, explain why and brainstorm
possible solutions.

NOTES 1:00 After my light lunch, I felt energized
to take a brisk walk around the block. I think I can
do that again tomorrow.

CURE FOR CRAVINGS

Did you use the daily cure for cravings to stick to your menu
plan? How did it work? Did you learn or do something that made
it easier for you to stick to your program today?

NOTES I realized that the sweet smells from
the bread and pastry shop that I pass on my
way home from work make me think about dessert
at the wrong time! Tomorrow I'll take a different
route home.

BIG BREAKFAST DIET

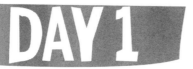

DATE:

MY WEIGHT
TODAY:

MY WAIST
TODAY:

MENU

MENU NOTES

BREAKFAST

LUNCH

DINNER

NOTES

> From small beginnings come great things.
> —*Proverb*

WORKOUT

Take a brisk 20-minute walk or perform one or two of the
10-minute workouts (chapter 8).

NOTES

CURE FOR CRAVINGS

Catch your cravings early. Many cravings awaken when you see or
smell the craved food (perhaps you walk by a doughnut shop or
pizza place); others when you think about them. The moment you
catch a craving rising, employ the tips in chapter 7 to nip it in the
bud. Before long, you'll recognize the situations that trigger your
cravings and be able to avoid them.

NOTES

BIG BREAKFAST DIET

DATE:

DAY 2

MENU

MENU NOTES

BREAKFAST

LUNCH

DINNER

NOTES

Do or do not. There is no try.

—*Yoda*

WORKOUT

Take a brisk 20-minute walk, or perform one or two of the
10-minute workouts (chapter 8).

NOTES

CURE FOR CRAVINGS

Shop in a square. When you go to the supermarket, avoid the
center aisles—that's where most of the junk foods are. Instead,
shop the perimeter of the store, where the dairy, bread, meat,
and produce sections are located.

NOTES

BIG BREAKFAST DIET

DATE: _____

DAY 3

MENU

MENU NOTES

BREAKFAST

LUNCH

DINNER

NOTES

> Start by doing what's necessary, then
> what's possible, and suddenly you are
> doing the impossible.
>
> —*Francis of Assisi*

WORKOUT

Take a brisk 20-minute walk or perform one or two of the
10-minute workouts (chapter 8).

NOTES

CURE FOR CRAVINGS

Drink a glass of one of the "free" beverages from page 65. Water
or club soda can protect your body from dehydration, which can
bring on fatigue, hunger, and food cravings.

NOTES

BIG BREAKFAST DIET

DATE: -

DAY 4

MENU

MENU NOTES

BREAKFAST

LUNCH

DINNER

NOTES

Don't let what you can't do interfere
with what you can do.

—*Anonymous*

WORKOUT

Take a brisk 20-minute walk or perform one or two of the
10-minute workouts (chapter 8).

NOTES

CURE FOR CRAVINGS

Save your shopping for Saturday or Sunday, after breakfast.
Your stomach will be full, and you're less likely to fill your
cart with unhealthy foods. Try to avoid shopping after work,
especially if you're prone to cravings in the late afternoon or
in the evening.

NOTES

BIG BREAKFAST DIET   DATE:

DAY 5

MENU

MENU NOTES

BREAKFAST

LUNCH

DINNER

NOTES

A jug fills drop by drop.

—*Buddha*

WORKOUT

Take a brisk 20-minute walk, or perform one or two of the 10-minute workouts (chapter 8).

NOTES

CURE FOR CRAVINGS

Keep your brain busy so your mouth won't be. When it's focused on the Sunday crossword puzzle, a computer game, or learning a new language on tape, your thoughts are less likely to turn to food.

NOTES

BIG BREAKFAST DIET   DATE:

DAY 6

MENU

MENU NOTES

BREAKFAST

LUNCH

DINNER

NOTES

You must do the thing you think you
cannot do.

—*Eleanor Roosevelt*

- -

WORKOUT

Take a brisk 20-minute walk, or perform one or two of the
10-minute workouts (chapter 8).

NOTES

- -

- -

- -

- -

- -

CURE FOR CRAVINGS

Don't set yourself up for failure. Diet "slips" happen for a reason,
and it's your job to figure out what that is. If you slip up, analyze
it. What happened? Did you skimp on your breakfast protein—or
did you skip breakfast entirely? Did you omit your breakfast
sweet to save a few calories, hoping to speed up your weight loss?
Once you figure out what went wrong, you can come up with a
way to keep it from happening again.

NOTES

- -

- -

- -

- -

- -

BIG BREAKFAST DIET

DATE:

DAY 7

MENU

MENU NOTES

BREAKFAST

LUNCH

DINNER

NOTES

Set your goals high, and don't stop till
you get there.

—*Bo Jackson*

WORKOUT

Take a brisk 20-minute walk, or perform one or two of the
10-minute workouts (chapter 8).

NOTES

CURE FOR CRAVINGS

Avoid temptation at work. If there is always candy and cake in
the break room, avoid that room during the day. If one of your
colleagues keeps a jar of candy on her desk, suck on a breath mint
when you stop by her office or cubicle to chat.

NOTES

BIG BREAKFAST DIET

DAY 8

DATE:
- - - - - - - - - - - - - - - - - - -

MY WEIGHT
TODAY:
- - - - - - - - - - - - - - - - - - -

MY WAIST
TODAY:
- - - - - - - - - - - - - - - - - - -

MENU

MENU NOTES

BREAKFAST

LUNCH

DINNER

NOTES

Motivation is what gets you started.
Habit is what keeps you going.

—Jim Ryun

WORKOUT

Take a brisk 20-minute walk, or perform two of the 10-minute workouts (chapter 8).

NOTES

CURE FOR CRAVINGS

Hide your breakfast sweets. The same goes for other starches or sweets you normally enjoy in the morning. You shouldn't crave these foods in the evening, but it's smart to keep them out of sight—in a high cupboard, for example.

NOTES

BIG BREAKFAST DIET

DAY 9

DATE:

MENU

MENU NOTES

BREAKFAST

LUNCH

DINNER

NOTES

People often say that motivation doesn't last. Well, neither does bathing—that's why we recommend it daily.

—*Zig Ziglar*

WORKOUT

Take a brisk 20-minute walk, or perform two of the 10-minute workouts (chapter 8).

NOTES

CURE FOR CRAVINGS

Wait out a craving. Research shows most cravings don't last more than ten minutes. So if one hits, delay that candy bar or dish of ice cream for at least that long. Then decide if you really want it. Chances are, you won't. (Or if you do, you won't mind saving it until tomorrow's breakfast.)

NOTES

BIG BREAKFAST DIET

DAY 10

DATE:

MENU

MENU NOTES

BREAKFAST

LUNCH

DINNER

NOTES

You may have to fight a battle more than once to win it.

—*Margaret Thatcher*

WORKOUT

Take a brisk 20-minute walk, or perform two of the 10-minute workouts (chapter 8).

NOTES

CURE FOR CRAVINGS

Cordon off your kitchen after dinner. A simple yet powerful tool to help you battle night eating: Tape a piece of string across the entrance to the kitchen.

NOTES

BIG BREAKFAST DIET   DATE:

DAY 11

MENU

MENU NOTES

BREAKFAST

LUNCH

DINNER

NOTES

Perseverance is failing nineteen times
and succeeding the twentieth.
—*Julie Andrews*

WORKOUT

Take a brisk 20-minute walk, or perform two of the 10-minute
workouts (chapter 8).

NOTES

CURE FOR CRAVINGS

Excuse-proof your routine. Develop a "Plan B" so that
unexpected events can't derail your diet. For example, keep some
sliced lean meat in the fridge at work in case a meeting runs long
and you don't have time to go out for lunch before the next one.

NOTES

BIG BREAKFAST DIET

DAY 12

DATE:

MENU

MENU NOTES

BREAKFAST

LUNCH

DINNER

NOTES

You will never plough a field if you only
turn it over in your mind.

—*Irish proverb*

WORKOUT

Take a brisk 20-minute walk, or perform two of the 10-minute
workouts (chapter 8).

NOTES

CURE FOR CRAVINGS

Use your hands when you watch TV. Hem a skirt, knit a sweater,
clip your dog's nails. When your hands are full, your mouth isn't.

NOTES

BIG BREAKFAST DIET

DATE:

DAY 13

MENU

	MENU NOTES
BREAKFAST	
LUNCH	
DINNER	

NOTES

> If you talk about it, it is a dream. If you plan it, it is possible. If you schedule it, it becomes reality.
>
> —*Anonymous*

WORKOUT

Take a brisk 20-minute walk, or perform two of the 10-minute workouts (chapter 8).

NOTES

CURE FOR CRAVINGS

Sip a glass of water. Sometimes when you have a craving for something sweet, you are simply dehydrated. Your craving may simply fade away.

NOTES

BIG BREAKFAST DIET

DATE:
- -

DAY 14

MENU

MENU NOTES

BREAKFAST

LUNCH

DINNER

NOTES

In the middle of difficulty lies
opportunity.

—Albert Einstein

WORKOUT

Take a brisk 20-minute walk, or perform two of the 10-minute
workouts (chapter 8).

NOTES

CURE FOR CRAVINGS

Brush your teeth. If you find yourself wandering into the kitchen
for a snack, head for the bathroom instead and pick up your
toothbrush. You'll freshen your breath, occupy your hands, and
snap yourself out of a craving.

NOTES

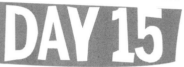

BIG BREAKFAST DIET

DATE:

MY WEIGHT
TODAY:

MY WAIST
TODAY:

MENU

	MENU NOTES
BREAKFAST	
LUNCH	
DINNER	

NOTES

"I can't do it" never yet accomplished
anything; "I will try" has performed
wonders.

—George P. Burnham

WORKOUT

If you feel ready to increase your workout, take a brisk
30-minute walk, or perform two or three of the 10-minute
workouts (chapter 8). If exercise is new to your lifestyle, stick
to the 20-minute workout from week 2.

NOTES

CURE FOR CRAVINGS

Don't label foods as "bad" or "forbidden." Remember, it's not
what you eat, but how much and when you eat it, that keeps
you overweight. As my plan proves, you can have some of all the
foods you love—if you time it right.

NOTES

BIG BREAKFAST DIET

DATE:

DAY 16

MENU

MENU NOTES

BREAKFAST

LUNCH

DINNER

NOTES

> We can do anything we want to do
> if we stick to it long enough.
>
> —*Helen Keller*

WORKOUT

Take a brisk 30-minute walk, or perform two or three of the
10-minute workouts (chapter 8). If exercise is new to your
lifestyle, stick to the 20-minute workout from week 2.

NOTES

CURE FOR CRAVINGS

Practice eating the foods you crave. If you're afraid to eat ice
cream or pizza because you can't stop once you start, try eating
them at breakfast. Eating them at the right time will likely tame
your out-of-control cravings for them.

NOTES

BIG BREAKFAST DIET   DATE:

DAY 17

MENU

MENU NOTES

BREAKFAST

LUNCH

DINNER

NOTES

Motivation is a fire from within. If
someone else tries to light that fire under
you, chances are it will burn very briefly.
—*Stephen R. Covey*

WORKOUT

Take a brisk 30-minute walk, or perform two or three of the
10-minute workouts (chapter 8). If exercise is new to your
lifestyle, stick to the 20-minute workout from week 2.

NOTES

CURE FOR CRAVINGS

Treat yourself. You've kept rigidly to the Turbocharged version of
the diet for more than two weeks. You deserve a reward. So treat
yourself—not with an ice-cream sundae (unless it's at breakfast),
but with a massage, a new lipstick, or a pedicure.

NOTES

BIG BREAKFAST DIET

DATE:

DAY 19

MENU

MENU NOTES

BREAKFAST

LUNCH

DINNER

NOTES

> The dictionary is the only place where
> success comes before work.
>
> —*Mark Twain*

WORKOUT

Take a brisk 30-minute walk, or perform two or three of the
10-minute workouts (chapter 8). If exercise is new to your
lifestyle, stick to the 20-minute workout from week 2.

NOTES

CURE FOR CRAVINGS

Be prepared for PMS cravings. Mark your calendar. To master
your cravings at "that time of the month," make sure to get
enough sleep, stay hydrated—and enjoy your breakfast sweet
without guilt.

NOTES

BIG BREAKFAST DIET

DATE:

DAY 20

MENU

MENU	MENU NOTES
BREAKFAST	
LUNCH	
DINNER	

NOTES

What would you attempt to do if you
knew you would not fail?
—*Robert Schuller*

WORKOUT

Take a brisk 30-minute walk, or perform two or three of the
10-minute workouts (chapter 8). If exercise is new to your
lifestyle, stick to the 20-minute workout from week 2.

NOTES

CURE FOR CRAVINGS

Ever heard of The Breakfast Club? Start a *Big* Breakfast club.
You're likely to find several neighbors and colleagues eager to join
you. Maybe members of your book group—or your family—are
interested in the diet. It's sometimes easier to stick to something
if your peers are committed to it, too.

NOTES

BIG BREAKFAST DIET

DATE:

DAY 21

MENU

MENU NOTES

BREAKFAST

LUNCH

DINNER

NOTES

Success usually comes to those who are
too busy to be looking for it.
—*Henry David Thoreau*

WORKOUT

Take a brisk 30-minute walk, or perform two or three of the
10-minute workouts (chapter 8). If exercise is new to your
lifestyle, stick to the 20-minute workout from week 2.

NOTES

CURE FOR CRAVINGS

Hang up on a craving. When all you can think of is chocolate-
chip cookies, pick up the phone and schedule an appointment or
discuss your bill with the electric company instead. You can call a
friend, too—but only if you can trust yourself not to munch while
you chat!

NOTES

BIG BREAKFAST DIET

DAY 22

DATE:
- -

MY WEIGHT
TODAY:
- -

MY WAIST
TODAY:
- -

MENU

MENU NOTES

BREAKFAST

LUNCH

DINNER

NOTES

> Do a little more each day than you think
> you possibly can.
>
> —*Lowell Thomas*

WORKOUT

If you feel ready to increase your workout again, take a brisk
40-minute walk, or perform three or four of the 10-minute
workouts (chapter 8). Otherwise, stick to the 20-minute workout
from week 2.

NOTES

CURE FOR CRAVINGS

Ask this question before you succumb to a craving: "Is this
[cookie, slice of pizza, whatever] more important right now
than meeting my goals?" Most of the time your answer will be
"no"—and simply deciding not to indulge a craving will help it
melt away.

NOTES

BIG BREAKFAST DIET

DATE:

DAY 23

MENU

MENU NOTES

BREAKFAST

LUNCH

DINNER

NOTES

Knowing is not enough; we must apply.
Willing is not enough; we must do.
—*Johann Wolfgang von Goethe*

WORKOUT

Take a brisk 40-minute walk, or perform three or four of
the 10-minute workouts (chapter 8). Otherwise, stick to the
20-minute workout from week 2.

NOTES

CURE FOR CRAVINGS

Keep busy during prime time. If you tend to snack in front of the
TV at night, first check out the list of Free Foods on page 65 and
snack on those. If you're all veggied out, find ways to distract
yourself during commercials. Instead of heading for the kitchen
during a commercial, check your e-mail, march in place, make
tomorrow's to-do list, or put in a load of laundry.

NOTES

BIG BREAKFAST DIET

DATE:
- -

DAY 24

MENU

MENU NOTES

BREAKFAST

LUNCH

DINNER

NOTES

The choices you make, make you.
—*Anonymous*

WORKOUT

Take a brisk 40-minute walk, or perform three or four of
the 10-minute workouts (chapter 8). Otherwise, stick to the
20-minute workout from week 2.

NOTES

CURE FOR CRAVINGS

Battle back from a binge. No matter how guilty you feel, eat
your next scheduled meal. For example, if you binged at night,
eat your normal breakfast—including your breakfast sweet. The
last thing you want is to starve yourself after a binge—the very
behavior that puts on extra pounds in the first place.

NOTES

BIG BREAKFAST DIET

DATE:

DAY 25

MENU

	MENU NOTES
BREAKFAST	
LUNCH	
DINNER	

NOTES

We are what we repeatedly do.
Excellence, therefore, is not an act
but a habit.

—Aristotle

WORKOUT

Take a brisk 40-minute walk, or perform three or four of
the 10-minute workouts (chapter 8). Otherwise, stick to the
20-minute workout from week 2.

NOTES

CURE FOR CRAVINGS

Do your cleaning on the weekends. Saturdays and Sundays
are packed with unstructured time, which can trigger boredom
eating. Tackle a large, messy project that involves your hands,
a bucket, and soap and water. Wash your car, scrub the kitchen
floor, and/or give your dog a much needed bath.

NOTES

BIG BREAKFAST DIET

DATE:

DAY 26

MENU

MENU NOTES

BREAKFAST

LUNCH

DINNER

NOTES

If you don't like something, change
it. If you can't change it, change your
attitude. Don't complain.

—*Maya Angelou*

WORKOUT

Take a brisk 40-minute walk, or perform three or four of
the 10-minute workouts (chapter 8). Otherwise, stick to the
20-minute workout from week 2.

NOTES

CURE FOR CRAVINGS

Chew gum while you cook. Many of you on my plan will still
have to get dinner on the table for your family even if you're
not hungry for it. To keep yourself from tasting or sampling as
you cook, pop a piece of sugarless chewing gum in your mouth.
Simple, but effective!

NOTES

BIG BREAKFAST DIET

DATE:

DAY 27

MENU

	MENU NOTES
BREAKFAST	
LUNCH	
DINNER	

NOTES

> The act of taking the first step is what
> separates the winners from the losers.
> —*Brian Tracy*

WORKOUT

Take a brisk 40-minute walk, or perform three or four of
the 10-minute workouts (chapter 8). Otherwise, stick to the
20-minute workout from week 2.

NOTES

CURE FOR CRAVINGS

Try something new. Is there a recipe you've always wanted to
try? Plan your next meal so it's fresh and exciting—even if you've
already identified meals that work for you, change it up. It might
be just what you need to keep making progress! (And while you're
at it, try something new for your workout, too: always wanted to
learn karate? cross-country skiing? boxing? Here's your chance.)

NOTES

BIG BREAKFAST DIET

DAY 28

DATE:

MY WEIGHT
TODAY:

MY WAIST
TODAY:

MENU

MENU NOTES

BREAKFAST

LUNCH

DINNER

NOTES

It's always fun to do the impossible.

—*Walt Disney*

WORKOUT

Take a brisk 40-minute walk, or perform three or four of
the 10-minute workouts (chapter 8). Otherwise, stick to the
20-minute workout from week 2.

NOTES

CURE FOR CRAVINGS

Leave the kids at home when you shop. Arrange for your spouse
or a friend to watch them when you go to the grocery store.
Without them begging you for junk, you'll find it easier to keep
to your shopping list and make healthy choices.

NOTES

SELECTED SCIENTIFIC REFERENCES

Affenito, S.G., Thompson, D.R., Barton, B.A., Franko, D.L., Daniels, S.R., Obarzanek, E., Schreiber, G.B. & Striegel-Moore, R.H. (2005). Breakfast consumption by African-American and White adolescent girls correlates positively with calcium and fiber intake and negatively with body mass index. *Journal of the American Dietetic Association, 105*(6), 938–45.

Avena, N.M., Rada, P. & Hoebel, B.G. (2008). Evidence for sugar addiction: behavioral and neurochemical effects of intermittent, excessive sugar intake. *Neuroscience & Biobehavioral Review, 32*(1), 20–39.

Baillargeon, J.P., Jakubowicz, D.J., Iuorno, M.J. & Nestler, J.E. (2004). Effects of Metformin and Rosiglitazone, alone and in combination, in non-obese women with polycystic ovary syndrome and normal indices of insulin sensitivity. *Fertility & Sterility, 82*(4), 893–902.

Barton, B.A., Eldridge, A.L., Thompson, D., Affenito, S.G., Striegel-Moore, R.H., Franko, D.L., Albertson, A.M. & Crockett, S.J. (2005). The relationship of breakfast and cereal consumption to nutrient intake and body mass index: The National Heart, Lung, and Blood Institute Growth and Health Study. *Journal of the American Dietetic Association, 105*(9), 1383–9.

Berkey, C.S., Rockett, H.R.H., Gillman, M.W., Field, A.E. & Colditz, G.A. (2003). Longitudinal study of skipping breakfast and weight change in adolescents. *International Journal of Obesity, 27,* 1258–66.

Berthoud, H.-R. & Morrison, C. (2008). The brain, appetite, and obesity. *Annual Review of Psychology, 59,* 55–92.

Blundell, J.E., Lawton, C.L., & Halford, J.C. (1995). Serotonin, eating behavior, and fat intake. *Obesity Research, 3* (Suppl 4), 471S–6S.

Bray, M.S. & Young, M.E. (2007). Circadian rhythms in the development of obesity: potential role for the circadian clock within the adipocyte. *Obesity Reviews, 8*(2), 169–81.

Carroll, S. & Dudfield, M. (2004). What is the relationship between exercise and metabolic abnormalities? A Review of the Metabolic Syndrome. *Sports Medicine, 34*(6), 371–418(48).

Castillo, M.R., Hochstetler, K.J., Tavernier Jr., R.J., Greene, D.M. & Bult-Ito, A. (2004) Entrainment of the master circadian clock by scheduled feeding. *American Journal of Physiology—Regulatory Integrative and Comparative Physiology, 287*(3), 551–5.

Chandler-Laney, P.C., Castaneda, E., Pritchett, C.E., Smith, M.L., Giddings, M., Artiga, A.I. & Boggiano, M.M. (2007). A history of caloric restriction induces neurochemical and behavioral changes in rats consistent with models of depression. *Pharmacology Biochemistry & Behavior, 87*(1), 104–14.

Cho, S., Dietrich, M., Brown, C.J., Clark, C.A. & Block, G. (2003). The effect of breakfast type on total daily energy intake and body mass index: results from the Third National Health and Nutrition Examination Survey (NHANES III). *Journal of the American College of Nutrition, 22*(4), 296–302.

Corwin, R.L. & Grigson, P.S. (2009). Symposium overview—Food addiction: fact or fiction? *Journal of Nutrition, 139*(3), 617–9.

De Castro, J.M. (2008). The time of day and the proportions of macronutrients eaten are related to total daily food intake. *British Journal of Nutrition, 98,* 1077–83.

Diamanti-Kandarakis, E., Baillargeon, J.P., Iuorno, M.J., Jakubowicz, D.J. & Nestler, J.E. (2003). A modern medical quandary: polycystic ovary syndrome, insulin resistance, and oral contraceptive pills. *Journal of Clinical Endocrinology & Metabolism, 88*(5), 1927–32.

Eng, S., Wagstaff, D.A. & Kranz, S. (2009). Eating late in the evening is associated with childhood obesity in some age groups but not in all children: the relationship between time of consumption and body weight status in U.S. children. *International Journal of Behavioral Nutrition & Physical Activity, 6,* 27.

Froy, O. (2007). The relationship between nutrition and circadian rhythms in mammals. *Frontiers in Neuroendocrinology, 28*(2-3), 61–71.

Gibson, S. (2003). Micronutrient intakes, micronutrient status, and lipid profiles among young people consuming different amounts of breakfast cereals: further analysis of data from the National Diet and Nutrition Survey of Young People aged 4 to 18 years. *Public Health Nutrition, 6,* 815–20.

Holt, S.H., Brand Miller, J.C. & Petocz, P. (1996). Interrelationships among postprandial satiety, glucose and insulin responses and changes in subsequent food intake. *European Journal of Clinical Nutrition, 50*(12), 788–97.

Iuorno, M.J., Jakubowicz, D.J., Baillargeon, J.P., Dillon, P., Gunn, R.D., Allan, G. & Nestler, J.E. (2002). Effects of d-*chiro*-inositol in lean women with the polycystic ovary syndrome. *Endocrine Practice, 8*(6), 417–23.

Jakubowicz, D.J. (2000). Insulin resistance in polycystic ovary syndrome. Medium and long term complications. *Médico Interamericano, 19*(9), 422–9.

Jakubowicz, D.J. & Sharma, S.T. (2007). "Insulin resistance and early pregnancy loss in polycystic ovary syndrome." In *Insulin Resistance and Polycystic Ovarian Syndrome: Pathogenesis, Evaluation, and Treatment (Contemporary Endocrinology)*, eds. Diamanti-Kandarakis, E., Nestler, J.E., Panidis, D. & Pasquali, R., 305–20. Totowa, NJ: Humana Press.

Jakubowicz, D.J., Beer, N.A., Beer, R.M. & Nestler, J.E. (1995). Disparate effects of weight reduction by diet on serum dehydroepiandrosterone-sulfate levels in obese men and women. *Journal of Clinical Endocrinology & Metabolism, 80,* 3373–76.

Jakubowicz, D.J., Beer, N. & Rengifo, R. (1995). Effect of dehydroepiandrosterone on cyclic-guanosine monophosphate in men of advancing age. *Annals of the New York Academy of Science, 774,* 312–5.

Jakubowicz, D.J., Maman, D. & Essah, P. (2008). Effect of diet with high carbohydrate and protein breakfast on weight loss and appetite in obese women with metabolic syndrome. *Endocrine News, 33*(7), 12.

Jakubowicz, D.J. & Nestler, J.E. (1997). 17α-hydroxyprogesterone response to leuprolide and serum androgens in obese women with and without polycystic ovary syndrome after dietary weight loss. *Journal of Clinical Endocrinology & Metabolism, 82,* 556–60.

Jakubowicz, D.J., Seppälä, M., Jakubowicz, S., Rodríguez-Armas, O., Rivas-Santiago, A., Koistinen, H., Koistinen, R. & Nestler, J.E. (2001). Insulin reduction with metformin increases luteal phase serum glycodelin and insulin-like growth factor-binding protein 1 concentrations and enhances uterine vascularity and blood flow in the polycystic ovary syndrome. *Journal of Clinical Endocrinology & Metabolism, 86*(3), 1126–33.

Kant, A.K., Andon, M.B., Angelopoulos, T.J. & Rippe, J.M. (2008). Association of breakfast energy density with diet quality and body mass index in American adults: National Health and Nutrition Examination Surveys, 1999–2004. *American Journal of Clinical Nutrition, 88*(5), 1396–404.

La Fleur, S.E. (2003). Daily rhythms in glucose metabolism: suprachiasmatic nucleus output to peripheral tissue. *Journal of Neuroendocrinology, 15*(3), 315–22.

Leibowitz, S. & Alexander, J. (1998). Hypothalamic serotonin in control of eating behavior, meal size, and body weight. *Biological Psychiatry, 44*(9), 851–64.

Lenard, N.R. & Berthoud, H.R. (2008). Central and peripheral regulation of food intake and physical activity: pathways and genes. *Obesity, 16,* 11–22.

Leproult, R., Colecchia, E.F., L'Hermite-Balériaux, M. & Van Cauter, E. (2001). Transition from dim to bright light in the morning induces an immediate elevation of cortisol levels. *Journal of Clinical Endocrinology & Metabolism, 86*(1), 151–7.

Levin, B.E. (2007). Why some of us get fat and what we can do about it. *Journal of Physiology, 583,* 425–30.

Lowden, A., Holmbäck, U., Åkerstedt, T., Forslund, A., Forslund, J. & Lennernäs, M. (2001). Time of day type of food-relation to mood and hunger during 24 hours of constant conditions. *Journal of Human Ergology, 30*(1–2), 381–6.

MacLean, P.S., Higgins, J.A., Johnson, G.C., Fleming-Elder, B.K., Peters, J.C. & Hill, J.O. (2004). Metabolic adjustments with the development, treatment, and recurrence of obesity. *American Journal of Physiology—Regulatory, Integrative & Comparative Physiology, 287,* 288–97.

Maffeis, C., Moghetti, P., Grezzani, A., Clementi, M., Gaudino, R. & Tato, L. (2002). Insulin resistance and the persistence of obesity from childhood into adulthood. *Journal of Clinical Endocrinology & Metabolism, 87*(1), 71–6.

Marshall, H.M., Allison, K.C., O'Reardon, J.P., Birketvedt, G. & Stunkard, A.J. (2004). Night eating syndrome among non-obese persons. *International Journal of Eating Disorders, 35*(2), 217–22.

McLaughlin, T., Allison, G., Abbasi, F., Lamendola, C. & Reaven, G. (2004). Prevalence of insulin resistance and associated cardiovascular disease risk factors among normal weight, overweight, and obese individuals. *Metabolism, 53*(4), 495–9.

Morgan, R., Paul, S.M. & Fisher, M.F. (2004). Challenges and strategies for proper pediatric nutrition and weight control. *New Jersey Medicine, 101*(5), 33–6.

Nestler, J.E., Beer, N.A., Jakubowicz, D.J., Colombo, C. & Beer, R.M. (1995). Effects of insulin reduction with benfluorex on serum dehydroepiandrosterone (DHEA), DHEA sulfate, and blood pressure in hypertensive middle-aged and elderly men. *Journal of Clinical Endocrinology & Metabolism, 80*(2), 700–6.

Nestler J.E. & Jakubowicz D.J. (1996). Decreases in ovarian cytochrome P450c17α activity and serum free testosterone after reduction of insulin secretion in women with the polycystic ovary syndrome. *New England Journal of Medicine, 335*(9), 617–23.

Nestler J.E. & Jakubowicz D.J. (1997). Lean women with polycystic ovary syndrome respond to insulin reduction with decreases in ovarian P450c17α activity and serum androgens. *Journal of Clinical Endocrinology & Metabolism, 82*(12), 4075–9.

Nestler, J.E., Jakubowicz, D.J., de Vargas, A.F., Brik, C., Quintero, N. & Medina, F. (1998). Insulin stimulates testosterone biosynthesis by human thecal cells from women with polycystic ovary syndrome by activating its own receptor and using inositolglycan mediators as the signal transduction system. *Journal of Clinical Endocrinology & Metabolism, 83*(6), 2001–5.

Nestler, J.E., Jakubowicz, D.J., Evans, W.S. & Pasquali, R. (1998). Effects of metformin on spontaneous and clomiphene-induced ovulation in the polycystic ovary syndrome. *New England Journal of Medicine, 338*(6), 1876–80.

Nestler, J.E., Jakubowicz D.J., Evans, W.S. & Pasquali R. (1998). Effects of metformin on spontaneous and clomiphene-induced ovulation in the polycystic ovary syndrome. *Obstetrical & Gynecological Survey, 53*(10), 621–2.

Nestler, J.E., Jakubowicz, D.J. & Iuorno, M.J. (2000). Role of inositolphosphoglycan mediators of insulin action in the polycystic ovary syndrome. *Journal of Pediatric Endocrinology & Metabolism, 13*(5), 1295–8.

Nestler, J.E., Jakubowicz, D.J., Reamer, P., Gunn, R.D. & Allan G. (1999). Ovulatory and metabolic effects of d-*chiro*-inositol in the polycystic ovary syndrome. *New England Journal of Medicine, 340*(17), 1314–20.

Nestler, J.E., Jakubowicz, D.J., Reamer, P., Gunn, R.D. & Allan, G. (1999). Ovulatory and metabolic effects of d-*chiro*-inositol in the polycystic ovary syndrome. *Obstetrical & Gynecological Survey,* *54*(9), 573–4.

Nestler, J.E., Stovall, D., Akhter, N., Iuorno, M.J. & Jakubowicz, D.J. (2002). Strategies for the use of insulin-sensitizing drugs to treat infertility in women with polycystic ovary syndrome. *Fertility & Sterility, 77*(2), 209–15.

Okosun, I.S., Dinesh Chandra, K.M., Boev, A., Boltri, J.M., Choi, S.T., Parish, D.C. & Dever, G.E. (2004). Abdominal adiposity in U.S. adults: prevalence and trends, 1960–2000. *Preventative Medicine, 39*(1), 197–206.

Perreau-Lenz, S., Pevet, P., Buijs, R.M. & Kalsbeek, A. (2004). The biological clock: the bodyguard of temporal homeostasis. *Chronobiology International, 21*(1), 1–25.

Radic, R., Nikolic, V., Karner, I., Kosovic, P., Kurbel, S., Selthofer, R. & Curkovic, M. (2003). Circadian rhythm of blood leptin level in obese and non-obese people. *Collegium Antropologicum, 27*(2), 555–61.

Rampersaud, G.C., Pereira, M.A., Girard, B.L., Adams, J. & Metzl, J.D. (2005). Breakfast habits, nutritional status, body weight, and academic performance in children and adolescents. *Journal of the American Diet Association, 105*(5), 743–60.

Reaven, G., Abbasi, F. & Mclaughlin, T. (2004). Obesity, insulin resistance, and cardiovascular disease. *Recent Progress in Hormone Research, 59,* 207–23.

Romon, M., Edme, J.L., Boulenguez, C., Lescroart, J.L. & Frimat, P. (1993). Circadian variation of diet-induced thermogenesis. *American Journal of Clinical Nutrition, 57*(4), 476–80.

Roseman, M.G., Yeung, W.K. & Nickelsen, J. (2007). Examination of weight status and dietary behaviors of middle school students in Kentucky. *Journal of the American Dietetic Association, 107*(7), 1139–45.

Scheen, A.J., Buxton, O.M., Jison, M., Van Reeth, O., Leproult, R., L'Hermite-Baleriaux, M. & Van Cauter, E. (1998). Effects of exercise on neuroendocrine secretions and glucose regulation at different times of day. *American Journal of Physiology, 274*(6), E1040–9.

Scheer, F.A., Hilton, M.F., Mantzoros, C.S., & Shea, S.A. (2009). Adverse metabolic and cardiovascular consequences of circadian misalignment. *Proceedings of the National Academy of Science USA, 106*(11), 4453–8.

Siega-Riz, A.M., Popkin, B.M. & Carson, T. (1998). Trends in breakfast consumption for children in the United States from 1965–1991. *American Journal of Clinical Nutrition, 67,* 748S–56S.

Slyper, A.H. (2004). The pediatric obesity epidemic: causes and controversies. *Journal of Clinical Endocrinology & Metabolism, 89*(6), 2540–7.

Smolenski, M. (2001). Circadian rhythms in medicine. *CNS Spectrums, 6*(6), 467–82.

Stanley, S., Wynnie, K., McGowan, B. & Bloom, S. (2005). Hormonal regulation of food intake. *Physiology Reviews, 85,* 1131–58.

Van Cauter, E. (2000). Slow wave sleep and release of growth hormone. *Journal of the American Medical Association, 284*(21), 2717–8.

Van Cauter, E., Blackman, J.D., Roland, D., Spire, J.P., Refetoff, S. & Polonsky, K.S. (1991). Modulation of glucose regulation and insulin secretion by circadian rhythmicity and sleep. *Journal of Clinical Investigations, 88*(3), 934–42.

Van Cauter, E., Polonsky, K. & Scheen, A. (1997). Roles of circadian rhythmicity and sleep in human glucose regulation. *Endocrine Review, 18*(5), 716–38.

Van der Heijden, A.W., Hu, F.B., Rimm, E.B. & van Dam, R.M. (2007). A prospective study of breakfast consumption and weight gain among U.S. men. *Obesity, 15,* 2463–9.

Weiss, R., Dziura, J., Burgert, T., Tamborlane, W., Taksali, S., Yeckel, C.W., Allen, K., Lopes, M., Savoye, M., Morrison, J., Sherwin, R.S. & Caprio, S. (2004). Obesity and the metabolic syndrome in children and adolescents. *New England Journal of Medicine, 350*(23), 2362–74.

Westerterp-Plantenga, M.S., Lejeune, M.P., Nijs, I., van Ooijen, M. & Kovacs, E.M. (2004). High protein intake sustains weight maintenance after body weight loss in humans. *International Journal of Obesity, 28,* 57–64.

Wolfe, W.S., Campbell, C.C., Frongillo, E.A. Jr., Haas, J.D. & Melnik, T.A. (1994). Overweight school children in New York State: prevalence and characteristics. *American Journal of Public Health, 84*(5), 807–13.

Wurtman, R.J. & Wurtman, J.J. (1995). Brain serotonin, carbohydrate-craving, obesity and depression. *Obesity Research, 3*(Suppl 4), 477S–80S.

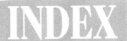

T

In memorium, to my parents

ACKNOWLEDGMENTS

With exceptional thanks to:

My sons, Salomon and Jonathan, and their wives, Karina and Claudine.

My grandson, Joshua.

My sister, Elizabeth, and her husband, Eli Zborowski.

My agents, Katherine Fausset and Matthew Guma, for never doubting the potential of this book.

My editor, Megan Nicolay, and everyone at Workman for making hard science accessible to the world.

My patients, for trusting me with their well-being for so many years.

ABOUT THE AUTHOR

DANIELA JAKUBOWICZ, M.D., is a specialist in endocrinology and metabolic diseases. She began her career at the Hospital de Clínicas Caracas in Venezuela. Since then, her work and presentations on metabolic syndrome and insulin resistance, obesity, diabetes, and infertility have taken her across the United States and to Israel, where she is now developing several related studies in conjunction with the Weizmann Institute of Science.

Dr. Jakubowicz's work has been published in some of the most respected scientific journals in her field, including *The Journal of Clinical Endocrinology & Metabolism*. She has also earned worldwide recognition for the honor of having three papers published in *The New England Journal of Medicine*.

Together with her mentor, Dr. John Nestler, Chairman of the Department of Endocrinology at Virginia Commonwealth University (where Dr. Jakubowicz is also a Professor of Medicine), she has published more than fifty studies on the effect of insulin resistance on obesity, polycystic ovary syndrome, and fertility. Through this work, and the Big Breakfast Diet she developed, Dr. Jakubowicz has served to radically change the way infertility, ovulation problems, and early pregnancy loss are prevented and treated. Her method not only has proven to treat obesity, but improve fertility, prevent diabetes and migraine, and reduce cardiovascular risk.

Dr. Jakubowicz currently lives and works in Israel.